# It Must Be My Hormones

*Getting your life on track with the help
of natural bio-identical hormone therapy
and nutrition*

DR MARION GLUCK *and*
VICKI EDGSON

MICHAEL JOSEPH
*an imprint of*
PENGUIN BOOKS

*Persons appearing in this book have had their names and identifying characteristics changed to protect their privacy*

MICHAEL JOSEPH

Published by the Penguin Group
Penguin Books Ltd, 80 Strand, London WC2R 0RL, England
Penguin Group (USA) Inc., 375 Hudson Street, New York, New York 10014, USA
Penguin Group (Canada), 90 Eglinton Avenue East, Suite 700, Toronto, Ontario, Canada M4P 2Y3
(a division of Pearson Penguin Canada Inc.)
Penguin Ireland, 25 St Stephen's Green, Dublin 2, Ireland (a division of Penguin Books Ltd)
Penguin Group (Australia), 250 Camberwell Road,
Camberwell, Victoria 3124, Australia (a division of Pearson Australia Group Pty Ltd)
Penguin Books India Pvt Ltd, 11 Community Centre, Panchsheel Park, New Delhi – 110 017, India
Penguin Group (NZ), 67 Apollo Drive, Rosedale, North Shore 0632, New Zealand
(a division of Pearson New Zealand Ltd)
Penguin Books (South Africa) (Pty) Ltd, 24 Sturdee Avenue, Rosebank, Johannesburg 2196, South Africa

Penguin Books Ltd, Registered Offices: 80 Strand, London WC2R 0RL, England

www.penguin.com

First published in Australia by Penguin Group (Australia) 2010
First published in Great Britain by Michael Joseph 2010

006

Text copyright © Marion Gluck and Vicki Edgson, 2010
Text design by Kirby Armstrong copyright © Penguin Group (Australia) 2010

The moral right of the authors has been asserted

**The information contained in this book is not intended as a substitute for consulting with your physician or other health care provider. The publisher and authors are not responsible for any adverse effects or consequences arising from the use of any suggestions, preparations or procedures contained in this book. All matters relating to your health should be discussed with your doctor.**

Printed in Great Britain by Clays Ltd, St Ives plc

A CIP catalogue record for this book is available from the British Library

ISBN: 978–0–718–15430–1

www.greenpenguin.co.uk

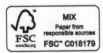

MIX
Paper from
responsible sources
FSC™ C018179
www.fsc.org

Penguin Books is committed to a sustainable
future for our business, our readers and our planet.
This book is made from Forest Stewardship
Council™ certified paper.

# contents

*Marion*: To all of my patients

*Vicki*: To my sister Shelley

# Acknowledgements

*Marion:* I would like to thank HRH Sultanah Kalsom for introducing me to Vicki; my friend Katja Krabiell, who let me stay in her pigeon tower in the Algarve while I was writing the first draft of the book; my cousin Daniel Topolski, who gave me the best advice a writer can get: 'just write; forget the grammar and punctuation'; and my son, Sam, who preferred not to know all the details about 'secret women's business'.

*Vicki:* My sincere thanks go to Kelly for sharing her beautiful cottage with us, in which both Marion and I wrote so studiously; to Amanda and Hugh for their beautiful home and stunning grounds, in which we surrounded ourselves with real nature and mammals that reminded us from whence we came; to Julie Gibb, Penguin Australia, who first commissioned this book several years ago; and to Louise Moore, Penguin UK, for picking it up from there, believing that this is an important book and running with it. Above all, thanks to Marion, who has illustrated beautifully how 'thinking outside the box' is vital in modern-day medicine, and without whom this book wouldn't be nearly as important as it is.

# introduction

Every day in my practice I encounter women who say they are feeling out of control, going crazy and losing a grip on their lives. Many of them are experiencing the extreme symptoms of menopause and side effects of conventional hormone replacement therapy (HRT). Others are suffering from the debilitating effects of postnatal depression, panic attacks, anxiety and other mood disorders. Many have suffered from endometriosis, cystitis or chronic infertility and are desperate for a solution and an end to their ordeal. And more and more women come to see me simply so that they can be well informed about the options out there as they go through hormonal changes, making them better prepared for life after menopause.

We know first hand what hormone hell is like – or we've seen our friends go through it and we want to avoid it for ourselves. This book is about your options as you negotiate the ups and downs of hormonal changes and the impacts these have on your life. Whether you are trying to fall pregnant, suffering from PMS, dealing with the post-pregnancy come-down, facing peri-menopause or the full-blown assault of menopause, you *do* have choices and a range of treatments *can* work.

Our Western medical environment is dominated by doctors who prescribe HRT or antidepressants and send women on their way. Few physicians are able or even willing to listen, then to 'join the dots' when it comes to the myriad of symptoms women experience as a result of hormonal imbalance, and then to offer a range of treatment options, from conventional drugs to bio-identical hormone therapy and alternative therapies.

Sometimes I find that patients do well with HRT and antidepressants; sometimes they do better on bio-identical hormones. And sometimes mine is not the only advice they need – they need the help of a nutritionist like Vicki, who can explain the powerful effects dietary changes can have on their hormone levels (more about Vicki's magical nutritional powers later).

Women often feel reduced to the role of a child when they visit their doctor, as if they need to take the doctor's advice 'or else'. I hope that this book will encourage you to be a proactive patient, to become a knowledgeable participant in your healthcare. Don't forget that you employ doctors to give you health advice; if you don't like their approach or methods, you can find someone else. The ideal is to find a doctor with whom you can work as a team focused on improving your health.

## THE POWER OF HORMONES

Hormones make us tick. They are the chemical messengers that continuously circulate in our bloodstream. They rule – and sometimes ruin – our lives. They regulate every function of the body, from building bone strength to helping us cope with stress. They are crucial to our ability to conceive and give birth, but hormones do much more than that.

Women go through a lifecycle of hormonal fluctuations, from puberty to menopause, sometimes with ease and at other times with major imbalances, which can lead to all the problems we know so well.

There are many treatment options for hormonal imbalances, the most common being HRT for menopause and, unfortunately, antidepressants for everything else. These drugs can be extremely effective when used appropriately, but they are not for everyone. There are usually better and healthier options, and many of my patients have found success using bio-identical hormone therapy if they are suffering the symptoms of hormonal withdrawal, as in menopause, or the hormonal imbalances that can occur at any stage of a woman's life.

## JUST WHAT IS BIO-IDENTICAL HORMONE THERAPY?

It sounds complicated and technical, but it's not. Bear with me. You really need to know about this.

Bio-identical hormones are derived from plant sources, such as soy beans and yams, and have an identical chemical structure to the hormones our body produces. They are identical to our own hormones in efficacy and we tolerate them in the same way. Of course, they are also natural – they already exist in nature.

The wonderful thing about these hormones is that the body recognises them as their own and they function as if the body had produced them itself. Another benefit of these hormones is that their combinations can be tailor-made specifically for each person's needs. These hormone preparations must be prescribed and monitored by a medical doctor (preferably your GP, who knows you best) and then made up in a compounding pharmacy, which specialises in compounding individual prescriptions. (For a more in-depth explanation of what bio-identical hormones are and how they work, see Chapter 2.)

Treating women with tailor-made bio-identical hormones is what I know best and enjoy most. And why shouldn't I? After treatment, my patients are more often than not healthy and happy. Many ask me, 'Why didn't anyone tell me about bio-identical hormones *before*?' You can read some of these patients' stories later in the book.

## THE POWER OF NUTRITIONAL CHANGES

That food and nutritional or herbal supplements can make a genuine difference to a woman's hormonal balance has been proven. You only have to look at the health of the inhabitants of Okinawa, an island off the coast of mainland Japan. For 25 years, researchers from the Harvard Medical School studied the diet and lifestyle of this population. What they found was that Okinawans had significantly lower rates of degenerative diseases compared to the Western world.

In Okinawa, the women never eat foods derived from cow's milk, favouring soy milk and other soy produce. They eat relatively low amounts of other animal products, except for fish and shellfish, of which there is an abundance surrounding their island. The women of Okinawa have virtually no hormone-related cancers, almost no heart disease and no obesity. They don't even have a Japanese word for the menopause, understanding the cessation of menstruation to be simply another phase in their lives. They live longer than almost any other peoples in the world.

There is now abundant research that illustrates the importance of supplementary minerals for bone health and density. As a woman matures, her digestive system becomes less efficient in breaking down and absorbing nutrients from her daily food, partly due to changes in hormonal balance. Eating calcium-rich foods is only part of the jigsaw puzzle, however; many co-factor nutrients are required to ensure the absorption of calcium by the bone, some of which are scarce in today's over-processed grains and greenhouse-grown vegetables.

Herbs such as clary sage, geranium, agnus castus and dong quai are all well-documented remedies for the relief of hot flushes, temper outbursts and other menopausal symptoms. Some work better than others for each individual, but all have proven to be effective in repeated trials.

Well-informed women are increasingly visiting clinics in search of 'natural remedies' that will allow them to take personal responsibility for their health as they mature. Weight management is still the greatest concern for most, as their metabolism and body-fat distribution change at the same time. Many dietary approaches have been touted, but the important point to understand is how *your* body works for *you*. The need for more protein and less carbohydrate in the menopausal years is now well understood medically, as is the fact that reduced calorie intake promotes healthy longevity. But a reduced calorie intake is only part of the story – which types of foods those calories are derived from is the other crucial issue.

In treating several thousand women in my clinic over the years, I have seen it all. In this book you will gain an insight – as I have – into how you can support your hormone balance by developing an eating program for life, rather than a short-term diet, to suit your own body type.

## OUR AIM

I never intended to write a book about hormone health, but during the 15 years that I have been specialising in the field, helping women get the balance back in their lives, I have met so many people who have said to me, 'Women *need* to know this!' So here's the book I wish had been around years ago.

In the pages that follow are the examples of 38 women and four men who have struggled with the effects of hormonal imbalance. We offer their stories, and the details of how they were treated, for you to see the options available and to inspire you to get the help you need.

We explain the role played by each of the major hormones in our body, how they work and why we need them. We hope that this information will explain why it is very common to sometimes feel out of control or like you are going crazy. Be assured that it is not your fault!

But before we proceed, Vicki and I would like to tell you our own stories – how we came to develop such a keen interest in the treatment of women with hormone problems.

Dr Marion Gluck and Vicki Edgson

# Marion's story

It wasn't until relatively late in my medical career that I became involved with hormones and women's health. It was only when I was working as a GP in Sydney that it even occurred to me to branch out into this exciting and relatively new field. How I came to be a pioneer in the area of bio-identical hormone replacement therapy is a long story, but along the way I learned a few valuable lessons. If you'll indulge me, I'll recount the ones that I think are most pertinent to the message of this book.

I earned my medical degree in Hamburg, Germany, where I went on to spend a turbulent year working in a hospital emergency room. These times were exhilarating, eye-opening and often disappointing. I loved the hype and adrenaline of it all; I loved the flurry of my white coat as I ran down the corridor into the emergency room, all eyes staring expectantly at my team and me. (Right now you are probably thinking about the television series *ER* or *Grey's Anatomy*. It wasn't quite as dramatic as that, but sometimes it got close.) I felt alive, vibrant and full of enthusiasm for my new profession and I felt powerful and in control – there is no time for wavering or indecision in an emergency.

It was between these times of stress and excitement, however, that I made my most profound discoveries. Saving lives was all well and good, but what came next? Unlike the heroes and heroines of *ER*, we emergency doctors were often required to be much more involved in our patients' recovery. We had to do more than just visit a patient once to say hello after they had made it to the ward.

When I was on my ward rounds, I noticed that the equipment we used for many procedures was invasive; I noted the adverse side effects of our recommended treatments and I observed that in many cases we caused pain to our patients. As doctors, we were always rushing from one patient to another, and so we never had much time to spend with each one. To them, we must have seemed cold and distant as we stood over their beds, glancing emotionlessly at our clipboards while prescribing drugs. These drugs had names that sounded like mythical lands: Xeloda, Imdur, Alimta, Ursofalk.

No wonder, then, that I often observed fear and misunderstanding as we walked past a patient's bed during ward rounds. We spoke about our charges in a language they couldn't understand and they were often too frightened or intimidated to ask questions. And of course it was at these times that they really needed to ask questions; they needed to speak up.

Being a patient should not be a passive experience. Medicine should not simply be something that *happens* to you; it should be something in which you take part – a collaboration of skills, ideas and beliefs. I always thought this, and yet it never occurred to me that others might not see it that way.

This revelation finally came as I consulted a patient who was to undergo surgery. It was a fairly minor operation, but there were a number of different ways to go about it, and I explained to him the procedures and potential side effects of each one. When I asked the man which procedure he wanted to undergo, he simply looked at me and said, 'You decide. You're the doctor.'

You may think that this was an understandable response, but I was deeply disappointed by it. We were, after all, talking about his body and his health, and yet he wanted someone else to make such a vital decision, to take responsibility for his wellbeing. I felt it was my job and my duty to make him understand his medical options, and thus give him the confidence to take an active part in his treatment. I was certainly responsible for his health, but I believed it was a shared responsibility. I was there to guide and advise him, to empower him even, but the *responsibility* of the decision was his. It was at this point that I realised something was wrong in this man's sense of helplessness, and that something was wrong with the medical system, which had rendered him so powerless in the face of this decision.

All patients should be aware that they are the subjects of a system that can cause harm just as easily as it can heal. Each patient should know, just as the public at large should know, that the third leading cause of death in all Western countries is iatrogenesis – a fancy term for 'medically induced adverse effects'. It's not that doctors harm their patients out of malice, or even stupidity – but the simple fact is that medicine is not the exact science you may always have thought it to be. The degree of biological variation between individuals is too great to guarantee that the same treatment will have the same effect on each patient.

My intention is not to scare you into avoiding hospitals or make you scream at the sight of white coats. Conventional medicine is still often your best option. In many cases it should be your first port of call, but under no circumstances should it be your only one. Furthermore, there is so much you can do to avoid having to undergo treatment in the first place. An apple a day on its own may not be enough to keep the doctor away, but a balanced, healthy diet that includes said apple could!

When reading this book, you should keep in mind a few important points.

1 You are not necessarily the same as that model skeleton or the fellow on the poster in your doctor's office who considerately shows you his innards – you are unique and, in most cases, it is to your advantage to find out how you differ from average.

2 I know we doctors tend to wear white robes, and some of us even have beards, but we are not gods. None of us is infallible.

3 Medical treatment is not something that 'happens to you' – it is something you take part in. That includes thinking about your health long before you even develop symptoms, making an informed choice about your treatment and whatever you do after treatment to stay well.

4 Hospitals are for those who couldn't avoid being ill, not for those who made themselves ill through laziness or neglect.

## OPENING MY EYES

As a young doctor in Germany I would occasionally trade the stress and excitement of the emergency room for the plodding predictability of a GP's office, where I would work as a locum. It was during this time that I became aware of the role of *Heilpraktiker*. These German healers-cum-naturopaths were not, unlike their colleagues in other developed countries, marvelled at and then belittled by patients as just another breed of strange fish in the medical sea. On the contrary, many German patients would see their *Heilpraktiker* even before they'd see their GP.

The fact that German patients regularly visited their naturopath didn't mean that they shunned conventional doctors, or that they blindly placed their faith in that one form of treatment. It just meant that they sought what they considered to be a more natural and less invasive solution. Naturopathy to them was not a replacement for conventional medicine as such, but rather provided another perspective on it.

By this time, I'd been exposed to the hospital environment long enough to become familiar with some of conventional medicine's biggest shortcomings. My first experiences of being a doctor were the medical profession's overly black-and-white approaches to decidedly grey problems. It began to irk me the way body parts were treated in isolation, with no consideration of the effects on other parts, as if they were all chopped up and organised neatly on a doctor's desk. Thus, curious and already somewhat disillusioned with the medical franchise as it was, I paid a great deal of attention to what those naturopaths were up to.

What I found was something that provided a fantastic complement to conventional medicine – a whole bunch of issues would be addressed while adding a pinch of that which is often sorely lacking in medicine: common sense. I had found myself on the path to *integrative and holistic medicine*.

This type of medicine is labelled 'integrative' because it feeds on the largest possible pool of medical knowledge. It combines the relatively new techniques of orthodox Western medicine with those of homeopathy or traditional Chinese medicine, whose proven efficacy does not come from wildly expensive, large-scale drug-company-funded studies, but from thousands of years of implementation and success. And it's called holistic because it considers the effects of treatments in terms of the entire body, rather than the body's isolated parts.

## THE ANTIPODEAN YEARS

With 10 years of medical experience behind me, I moved to Sydney, Australia, where my family lived, and where I wanted my son to grow up. Here, I experienced yet another unsavoury side to the medical fraternity, of which I was increasingly reluctantly a part. Despite the fact that I was an Australian citizen, the Australian medical board saw fit not to recognise my German medical degree.

In response to this, I threw down my stethoscope and took up the role of activist. I became president of the Australian Doctors Trained Overseas Association, which lobbies the government and medical groups on behalf of doctors who live in Australia but have been denied the right to practise. After four busy – and sometimes dispiriting – years as a medical activist, I finally swallowed my pride, sat for the Australian medical council exams and won back my right to practise the profession that I had been trained, if not born, for.

My not-so-brief stint in politics had, however, left its indelible mark, and I like to think that some of the passion that saw me lobbying for the rights of overseas-trained doctors transferred itself to a passion for pioneering a better way of practising medicine.

As a GP in Australia, I gained a good reputation through my individual approach to my patients and the integrative, holistic treatments that I offered. In the early 1990s, women in increasing numbers began coming to me for help in getting off their hormone replacement therapies.

This was a time when the slogan 'hormones for all women for the rest of their lives' was on the tip of every doctor's tongue – and probably on their bumper stickers too. Merely being over the age of 45 was often a good enough excuse to be put on HRT. The pharmaceutical companies that produced synthetic hormones were marketing them as preventative drugs, ones that decreased the chance of stroke, heart disease and osteoporosis. All women, they insisted, should be put on synthetic hormones as soon as they started experiencing the hormonal fluctuations that often herald the onset of menopause.

Women on conventional HRT were coming to me because, in their own words, they 'weren't feeling right' or 'weren't feeling like themselves'. They came to me complaining of weight gain and increased breast size, as well as a lack of motivation, energy and libido. The women were also becoming aware of the then still emerging reports of the possible increased risk of cancer – breast cancer in particular – associated with the use of synthetic hormones. These reports, when they appeared in the media, were often played down by doctors who offered conventional hormone treatments, while others admitted that the risks may very well have been real, but that the benefits of conventional HRT far outweighed them.

Today, we know from the 2002 Women's Health Initiative (WHI) study how wrong these statements were. The ethics committee in charge of this study had to halt the trials prematurely because of the *increased* risk of stroke, heart disease and breast cancer in the group of women who were on combined synthetic HRT.

This emphasised to the public the dangers and risks incurred in taking synthetic hormones such as Premarin and Provera (more about this later). It also highlighted the importance of the *right* hormones in the *right* balance for women, and by the right hormones I mean those agents that are naturally found in the human body: oestradiol, oestriol, progesterone and testosterone. How each of these hormones operates will be explained in detail later in this book.

I became known as a doctor who could wean women off synthetic hormones, helping them over the hump with a combination of natural therapies, nutritional advice, supplements, vitamins and lifestyle changes. For many patients, this was enough, but there were others whose symptoms returned when they stopped their HRT, and there were even those who couldn't cope without HRT and had to return to it, albeit reluctantly. HRT, I realised, was necessary for many patients.

The challenge was to find a form of HRT that, rather than rudely upsetting the body's natural balance, merely fine-tuned it. What I needed was a therapy that was the equivalent of gently placing a finger on the endocrine scale, as opposed to smacking it off the table, which is what conventional HRT and synthetic hormones often manage to do.

I began offering hormone-replacement therapies using only bio-identical hormones (oestradiol, oestriol, progesterone and so on) with the exact amounts of hormones, and the ratios between them, individually tailored to each patient.

It was the *balance* of hormones, I realised, that made all the difference. Doctors needed to solve each patient's endocrine puzzle before they could even begin to prescribe hormones. Too much oestrogen, too little progesterone – every undersupply or oversupply of a hormone, no matter how minute, meant a different approach. Hormones, after all, regulate every function of our body, from intellect to energy, from mood to metabolism. The previously ham-fisted attempts of doctors (and pharmaceutical companies) to introduce large amounts of synthetic hormones into these intricately balanced systems were like trying to perform surgery with a mallet.

Today, modern, health-conscious women and men are taking control, are more informed and are requesting natural solutions for a natural change in their lives. This book provides you with the information you need about bio-identical hormones, nutrition and lifestyle choices to empower you to make your own decisions and take control of your life.

# Vicki's story

As a woman hurtling into peri-menopause at the speed of a super-fast train, I have a vested interest in efficiently and safely managing the frightening array of physical and psychological changes that come with this transition. You might think that as a practising nutritionist and naturopath I would know *exactly* how to handle this situation, but life has an extraordinary habit of 'getting in the way'.

Meeting Dr Marion Gluck in Australia some five years ago was a revelation for me. I had many patients either heading towards or already experiencing menopause, and Marion ultimately made a big impact on how I came to treat them. When we met, we found that we were *simpatico* and cared deeply about the same issues. We agreed that there would be a time when we would work together, but Marion was firmly fixed in Australia at that time, while I was living in the UK.

We kept in touch through mutual patients and friends. That we should write a book together was obvious. We are women of the same age – one a mother (Marion) and the other childless (me: more about this later) – and are both dedicated to the pursuit of health, knowledge, taking responsibility for our own lives and to showing others how to do the same.

But aside from my experience as a health practitioner, I write as a woman who has been the patient of many doctors, gynaecologists, fertility specialists and holistic practitioners over the years. My journey into womanhood has been very different from how I envisaged it in my teens, and I bring to this book a great understanding of the frustrations, fears, pain and disappointments that many women suffer.

My menarche (first period) occurred when I was nearly 14 – late by all standards, which was hugely frustrating to a girl locked in the competitive frenzy of boarding school. The pain was excruciating, way beyond any level that my mother had prepared me for. This was no 'dull ache in the lower abdomen' – it was more like wrenching knives. I felt sick and listless for four days, and spent the first two in bed, doubled up in pain, with only an aspirin from Matron every six hours. It was hell.

I continued to suffer like this every month for nearly a year before telling my mother. She immediately took me to her gynaecologist, who announced that I probably had a 'narrow neck to the cervix' and promptly booked me in for the insertion of an IUD – the subsequently banned Dalkon Shield. For several months after this minor procedure, I suffered far less on a monthly basis, and thought 'that was that'.

I got pregnant at 18, barely a year after my mother had died. My father organised a termination with military precision, concealing his shame and disbelief behind his need to hold the family together. As I lay on the gurney, waiting to go into the operating theatre, I saw a woman come out of that same theatre, sobbing and crying, 'I shouldn't have done it.' I'll never forget her voice; it came from the very pit of her womb. My procedure went 'smoothly', although I was informed that the Dalkon Shield would have to be removed as it had 'become embedded in the wall of your uterus, which is probably why it wasn't effective in preventing you from getting pregnant'. A little extra surgery to remove that offensive device and I would be fine.

I wasn't – I continued to bleed extremely heavily every month, with clots that seemed the size of my liver. I dreaded that time of month. Don't get me wrong, though, I didn't loathe my body. I loved sex and adored men, and had some wonderful partners through-out those years. I tried several different IUD devices, including the Copper 7, which turned me into a 'bitch from hell'. It's only now that I realise how highly sensitive I was to these devices being inserted into my body. Eventually my GP advised me to go on the contracep-tive pill, which I duly did.

I fell pregnant again (while on the pill), and felt it almost imme-diately, as I had become finely attuned to my bodily changes. I went for no fewer than five pregnancy tests, always to be told that I wasn't pregnant, until, finally, at 12 weeks a new gynaecologist confirmed that indeed I was. My heart sank – the potential father couldn't have been more unsuitable as a long-term partner; at the time he was battling with drug addiction and alcoholism. I wasn't ready to be a single mother. I went ahead with a second termination.

While the clinical procedure went smoothly, my mind was in turmoil. I couldn't walk on the same side of the road as a woman pushing a pram, and I had to leave a coffee shop if anyone walked in with a young child. I felt like a murderer and crucified myself for my decision. Time is a great healer, though, and I gradually came to terms with the fact that I was still young, and that there would be plenty of time to have children with the right man.

That man came into my life when I was in my 30s, in the form of someone who already had a child of his own, was some 10 years my senior, and knew what he wanted in life, which included more children. We started to try for a pregnancy.

After a year or so, I went to my gynaecologist to have a full hor-monal screening to check that 'there was nothing wrong'. There wasn't, apparently, but my husband and I still thought it wise to get 'super-healthy' – both of us stopped drinking alcohol, went to the gym four evenings a week and ate fantastically healthy food.

After three years of trying, my gynaecologist referred me to a leading fertility expert in London. I was nearly 40, and my time was running out. The fertility specialist put me on a cocktail of hormones to 'move me forward'. I insisted that the nurse teach me how to self-administer the daily injections, to help stem the endless hours spent waiting in the hospital for an available nurse.

I hated the hormones. I became depressed, argumentative and volatile – this was so far removed from the person I really was. I also had concerns about my marriage: there was intense pressure on my husband to 'perform at the right time' and on me to get a positive result each month. The whole process was turning into a nightmare.

And so, much against my inclination, we tried IVF. My husband was away at the time, so his sperm had to be frozen. This, of course, wasn't ideal, but there was nothing else we could do. Around that time I remember calling my sister from the bridge over the Serpentine in London and telling her I was about to jump, to which she responded, 'Well, if you're going to jump, Vick, I would suggest you try a higher bridge.' Her humour made me climb down, but I realised that the hormones I was taking were having a major effect on my sanity. I made a promise to myself that I'd go through IVF once, but that they'd have to lock me up before I went through it again.

It didn't work. I decided that if I were meant to have a child, I would get pregnant naturally, but I would not take any more hormones. I loved the other aspects of my life and something told me that maybe I wasn't meant to have children anyway – a belief I eventually came to feel in my heart and not just in my head. Several years later my husband and I divorced, thankfully for reasons other than not having been able to have a child together.

It was during those years of trying for a baby that I came to discover not just how potent hormones can be for a person's health, but also how nutrition can make such a powerful difference. Towards the end of my 20s I had developed fairly serious and frequent migraines. I knew these weren't hormonally related, because they would occur without rhyme or reason and usually in clusters of three or four within a couple of weeks. A friend sent me to her doctor, Guy Staight in Chelsea, saying she just knew he would sort me out – that he would look at the big picture. I shall be indebted to Guy forever. He recognised that I had classic food-intolerance migraines, identifying caffeine, dairy foods and chocolate as my major triggers. I went on a total caffeine-, dairy- and chocolate-free diet for a year after seeing him and, amazingly, suffered only one headache during that whole time.

Needless to say, I was hooked. I couldn't believe that foods, either included or omitted from a person's diet, could have such a profound effect on their health. I immediately sought out all the nutrition colleges in London.

I studied at the Institute for Optimum Nutrition, adding in a year of biochemistry at another college when I had attained my diploma in Nutrition Consultancy, and a further two years' naturopathic studies on a post-graduate basis once I had set up my own clinic. From the outset, I was fortunate to meet many doctors, gastroenterologists and psychiatrists who shared my belief that complementary medicine could run alongside conventional medicine to create a better outcome for patients. Many of these doctors have been referring their patients to me ever since.

I met my business partner, Ian Marber, three years after I set up in practice, and together we co-authored *The Food Doctor: Healing Foods for Mind and Body*, in 1997. It has sold well over a million copies and been translated into 10 languages. Such was the success of the book that we shortly thereafter set up a clinic and a business with the same name, in the belief that we should take the message of good nutrition to every man, woman and child in the UK, rather than keeping the knowledge of balanced nutrition and diet for the fortunate few. Together, we designed a range of foods for one of the leading supermarket chains, set up nutrition practices in many of the premier banking and other corporate communities, and eventually created a household brand within Britain. I wrote two more books under the Food Doctor label: *In Bed with the Food Doctor* and *The Food Doctor for Babies and Children*.

But as the responsibilities of running a large business took their toll, I found I was frustrated not to be more available to work as a nutrition consultant on a day-to-day basis. I became particularly interested in working with autistic children, so I resigned from the company and worked alongside medical practitioners in a thrilling and extremely rewarding area. I should say explicitly, though, that I don't believe nutrition is the only answer to autism; it can, however, help enormously with some of the more rudimentary daily problems that children with autism can suffer.

At this point, I also became involved with the BBC television series *Fat Nation*. This was followed by *The Diet Doctors: Inside and Out*, which I co-presented with Dr Wendy Denning. The series was accompanied by a book of the same title and was as successful as the first *Food Doctor* book.

My present-day activities find me working in my own busy clinic, part of the time in association with Marion and part of the time with other health practitioners, while I am also involved with spa and retreat companies, and do some writing for magazines and newspapers.

I am a lucky woman. I have had such a rewarding time helping others through my nutritional consultancy. And I have plenty of children in my life, so that I no longer have any regrets about not having my own. My wonderful sister has two beautiful children, whom she has shared with me and allowed me to take pleasure in as though they were my own. I have 12 godchildren all over the world.

But my experiences have all equipped me with a greater understanding of just how frightening, frustrating and isolating these types of female problems can be. My use of synthetic hormones has taught me just how mind-altering they can be, not to mention the physical challenges they can give rise to. I have experienced the weight gain, the fluid retention, the unsightly thread veins in the legs, the blinding headaches, the ringing in the ears – all of which the doctors and specialists had warned me I 'might experience a little of'.

My work with Marion has shown how highly sensitive I am to hormones. All people are individuals – there is no 'one size fits all' approach to dealing with hormones, just as there isn't one for nutritional needs.

Having battled the most furious hormonal havoc throughout my adult life, I cannot stress enough how enlightening and empowering it is to understand fully how your body works and what you can give it to perform optimally. The correct hormones in the right balance for *you* will have you feeling better than you have felt for years. Adding the correct nutrition, herbal remedies and ancient practices of relaxation and exercise will have you feeling phenomenal. At 50, I feel better than I felt at 30, and I can't ask for more than that.

If you've bought this book, then you are seeking solutions to hormonal issues you may be aware of or simply suspect. I suggest you take the day off, curl up on the sofa and allow yourself the time to digest what Marion and I have brought together for this book. I promise you, it will be worth it.

# 1

# the politics of menopause

## THE SOCIAL CONTEXT OF MENOPAUSE

Menopause is not simply a biological event. It is more than just that stage in a woman's life when menstruation ceases. Rather, it is inextricably tied to our social history, to changes in medical science, to legal reform, to feminism and to politics. It is important that all women have a sense of how menopause and hormones have been viewed throughout history. You may be surprised by how much we take for granted.

To put menopause in context we need to look at the wider issues of birth control and women's rights. The emancipation of women is closely related to access to contraception.

Throughout history the responsibility of child-rearing – as well as for birth control – has largely fallen to women. Since ancient times many (mainly unreliable) contraceptive methods have been used, from *coitus interruptus*, to douching, vaginal suppositories made of acidic substances, and herbal remedies to induce miscarriage. Even in Casanova's 18th-century memoirs, there are descriptions of attempts to use the empty rind of half a lemon as a primi-tive cervical cap. Although condoms had been around in various forms – including linen sheaths and animal intestines – it wasn't until the industrial age that contraceptive equipment was produced on a large scale. In 1844, American manufacturer Charles Goodyear started to mass-produce condoms, douching devices and 'womb veils' made from vulcanised rubber. By the late 19th century, a large assortment of birth-control devices was available in most Western countries. These included condoms, sponges, douching syringes, cervical caps and diaphragms, most of which could be found in catalogues, pharmacies and dry-goods stores.

Though the responsibility of contraception has fallen mainly to women, some did not have the right to practise it until relatively recently. In 1873, the US Congress passed the Comstock Law, an anti-obscenity act that specifically listed contraceptive devices as obscene and outlawed their commerce. Documents relating to reproductive information were also banned. The US was the only Western nation to enact laws criminalising birth control. It was not until 1965 that this law was revoked in all American states.

The phrase 'birth control' was coined by Margaret Sanger (1879–1966), an obstetric nurse who had been charged under the Comstock Law for distributing information about contraception. She vowed to see the Comstock Law repealed and wanted to ensure that all women had access to contraceptive information and counselling; she even dreamt of a 'magic pill' that could one day be used to control reproduction. Sanger went on to play a further role in the history of contraception, but more on that later. During her lifetime, she bore witness to some momentous events. The suffragette movement took hold and women in various Western nations won the right to vote; women's voices were starting to be heard in political and social arenas. Having their voices heard in the resolutely male-dominated world of medicine was the next frontier.

## THE HISTORY OF MENOPAUSE

The term 'menopause' was first used by French physician Charles de Gardanne in 1812. It comes from the Greek word *mens*, meaning 'monthly', and *pausus*, meaning 'cessation'. De Gardanne described it as 'the critical age for women'. Around this time menopause was not really on anyone's agenda. This is not as surprising as it might seem: in the 19th century the majority of women were either pregnant or lactating, and most bore between 10 and 14 pregnancies over their lifespan. A woman's life expectancy sat below the age of 50, and the cause of death was often childbirth. Most women never experienced the effects of menopause because they never reached this 'critical age'.

With the 20th century and the huge advances in technology, medicine and infection control that came with it, the life expectancy of women increased. The first half of the 20th century, however, saw men and women the world over struggling to meet other challenges – with two world wars and the Great Depression, these were about survival. Although women were living longer, hormonal problems and menopause were non-issues. Women did not have the luxury to indulge themselves while men were at war or while trying to carve out a new existence for their families in the post-war years.

## THE DISCOVERY OF SEX HORMONES

The 1930s were a vital decade in the history of hormones. A new class of steroid hormones was discovered during this time. Of these, progesterone was the most interesting because it was a precursor – that is, an essential building block – in the production of another class of exciting new steroid hormones, the glucocorticoids. Glucocorticoids, which occur naturally in the human adrenal gland, are vital for life and instrumental in controlling many of our body's metabolic processes.

One such glucocorticoid, cortisol, proved lifesaving for John F. Kennedy. It is possible that he would have never survived to become president had it not been discovered. Kennedy suffered from Addison's disease, meaning that his adrenal glands did not produce the hormone cortisol, which the body requires to regulate such vital functions as blood pressure, the immune system and the fight-or-flight response.

The potential of these hormones was not lost on the medical establishment. For his discovery of adrenal cortex hormones, as well as their structures and functions, Edward Calvin Kendall was awarded the Nobel Prize in Physiology or Medicine in 1950. These steroid hormones represented a powerful new tool in the fight against disease, acting as potent anti-inflammatory agents and immune suppressants.

In the early days the production of these hormones, specifically progesterone, was not economically feasible, and research and development efforts were often thwarted. In 1934, Schering Laboratories managed to isolate just 20 grams of progesterone from the ovaries of 50000 sows!

Natural progesterone therapy required huge doses to be effective, and at a cost of anywhere from US$80 to $100 per gram, only the richest patients could afford the treatment. In fact, the only customers for natural progesterone were world-class horse breeders, who used it to improve the fertility of their mares. They knew when they were onto a good thing and were willing to pay for it.

## FROM SARSAPARILLA TO PROGESTERONE

In 1904, Katherine McCormick was the first woman to graduate from the Massachusetts Institute of Technology with a degree in science. In 1906, her husband was diagnosed with schizophrenia and Katherine was convinced that the disease was hereditary. She vowed never to have children and became a staunch supporter of contraception. In 1917, McCormick met our old friend Margaret Sanger at one of Sanger's lectures on birth control. This started a long-lasting friendship. McCormick supported Sanger's work and later helped to finance research into hormones, in particular the work of a chemist called Russell Earl Marker.

Marker was an ingenious, unique and eccentric chemist. He was convinced that the plant kingdom was the place to look for abundant, inexpensive raw materials for steroids. In 1938, he developed a hypothesis that contradicted all prevailing chemical beliefs: if atoms were removed from the side chain of the molecular structure of sarsasapogenin, a steroid from the sarsaparilla plant (which we use today as soft-drink flavouring), this would convert it into progesterone. Sarsaparilla was an extremely expensive material at the time, however, and Marker was forced to find a less expensive chemical relative of sarsasapogenin. He searched the woodlands from Canada to Mexico, and finally found what he was looking for in *Dioscorea mexicana* – a wild yam native to the east coast of Mexico.

He puzzled over the precise molecular structure of many sapogenins (plant steroids) and eventually devised a method, which he coined the 'Marker degradation process', for converting plant steroids (sapogenins) into human steroids (progesterone). Marker took this breakthrough to two large American pharmaceutical companies, but they deemed mass production too risky. They could not imagine the use of natural progesterone as a means of contraception.

In 1949, disappointed by the lack of interest in his discoveries, Marker retired from chemical research. He never patented his discovery and it fell into the public realm – which of course meant that, down the track, once pharmaceutical companies realised that Marker had been onto something, they were able to make their own hormones in a pill form and then patent them as their own invention. The first oral contraceptive pill – the 'magic pill' that Sanger had so desired to see – was developed in the 1950s.

Marker's discovery was only one breakthrough on the way to developing an effective oral contraceptive. There were still many hindrances to overcome. In the early 1950s, the obstructions to the emergence of the pill were both scientific and political. Although the Marker degradation process provided a means of producing progesterone cheaply, the only method of delivery at that time was via injection, which was painful and inefficient. Furthermore, the Comstock Law still restricted the sale of contraceptives in 30 US states and it was expected that Catholics, who represented roughly a quarter of the population, would boycott any mass-produced contraceptive. As a result, most pharmaceutical companies remained unwilling to fund research into contraceptives.

It was by accident, then, that Frank Colton, a researcher working for the pharmaceutical company G. D. Searle, developed a synthetic progesterone compound that was effective orally. Colton, among other Searle researchers, was looking into various steroids in the hope of finding the next miracle drug. As it happened, Colton's synthetic progesterone compound, known as norethynodrel, worked as an effective anti-ovulent. Searle was naturally unwilling to fund the development of the oral contraceptive and instead let a scientist from outside, Gregory Pincus, conduct the trials. This allowed Searle to distance itself from the political risk that the tests entailed.

When Searle first released the pill, under the brand name Enovid, in 1957, it was marketed as a medication for the treatment of gynaecological disorders. However, women began increasingly to use it for its off-label purpose – birth control. In 1960 the FDA finally approved Enovid for contraceptive use.

## THE MEDICALISATION OF MENOPAUSE

In the 1950s and 1960s, with the beginnings of the women's liberation movement, women became more vocal about their sexuality and their physical needs and concerns. Contraception became a huge issue, and the taboo surrounding birth control slowly started to break down.

Even at the beginning of the women's movement, menopause was still regarded as an embarrassing problem, and women were reluctant to discuss it. Nevertheless, women in their 40s and 50s started going to their doctors complaining of symptoms as diverse as anxiety, fatigue, panic attacks, agoraphobia, insomnia, night sweats, hot flushes, depression, migraines and weight gain.

These symptoms were regarded as part of a natural passage in a woman's life, and often she was advised to grin and bear it, just as her mother and grandmother had done before her. The only treatment women were likely to receive was a sedative, such as Valium, or an antidepressant. Women were going through nervous breakdowns and no one really questioned why.

In 1966, Dr Robert Wilson, an American gynaecologist, wrote a book called *Feminine Forever*, which called menopause 'an oestrogen-deficiency disease'. Wilson proclaimed that oestrogen, in the form of Premarin, was the 'new fountain of youth'. Premarin is a product made from the oestradiol-rich urine of pregnant mares (see page 35 for more about the history of this drug). Premarin promised women the chance to 'remain fully feminine, physically and emotionally, for as long as they live', and to avoid the scourges of old age, such as shrivelling skin and brittle bones.

Wilson expressed his 'sympathy' to women who were 'condemned to witness the death of their own womanhood'; he referred to himself as the 'gallant knight' on a mission to help women. Wilson lauded the medical breakthrough that allowed us 'the opportunity to remain complete women'. With the backing of a major pharmaceutical company and without the necessary research into side effects, the great Premarin experiment began. Ten years after the publication of *Feminine Forever*, Premarin was the fifth leading prescription drug in America.

## WOMEN AS GUINEA PIGS

It didn't take long for studies to show an increase in cases of uterine cancer in women who were taking Premarin by itself (or 'unopposed' by progesterone). Premarin increases the thickness of the lining of the uterus – this is what we call endometrial hyperplasia and it is a risk factor for cancer of the womb.

At around the same time as these discoveries were taking place, in the late 1960s, a generation of women was being prescribed the oral contraceptive pill. Although the women's liberation movement lauded the newfound freedom that came with this, it also became increasingly critical of the drug companies supplying the pill. The movement accused these companies of deliberately withholding information about side effects, such as increased risk of uterine and breast cancer and stroke, high blood pressure, blood clots, hair loss, depression and birth defects.

By 1972, there was a moratorium on the unopposed use of Premarin (or any other oestrogen) to treat menopause. The public was made aware of the dangers related to the use of synthetic hormones and the sales of Premarin as oestrogen-replacement therapy (ERT) plummeted. Research into oral contraceptives continued at the same time, and a new generation of the pill, with much lower dosages of oestrogen and progesterone, was introduced.

## 'HORMONES FOR ALL WOMEN FOR THE REST OF THEIR LIVES'

The pharmaceutical companies' favourite drug had fallen into disrepute, but they were hesitant to give it up for dead. The massive popularity of the pill had normalised the use of hormones among women, the medical fraternity and the media. Women were living much longer and there was a huge market for the taking – women who had become increasingly outspoken about their menopausal symptoms and wanted relief.

The pharmaceutical industry pushed to find a way to restore Premarin's good name. Women between the ages of 40 and 60 were all considered to be afflicted with 'oestrogen-deficiency syndrome' and the perception of menopause changed. It was no longer just an end of menstruation or a 'change in life'; it was now a deficiency disease or an 'illness'. Like diabetes, it required medical treatment.

Research showed that taking Premarin in combination with a synthetic version of progesterone (a progestogen) decreased the incidence of uterine cancer. This was a great relief for all. Other research indicated that the newly coined 'hormone-replacement therapy (HRT)', in the form of Premarin and Provera (a progestogen), prevented osteoporosis, colon cancer, and apparently stroke and heart disease too, while also reducing all the menacing effects of menopause from which many women suffered. What a bonanza!

With HRT packaged as 'preventative medicine', pharmaceutical companies lobbied doctors, the media followed uncritically, and HRT (no longer ERT) was viewed as a panacea. 'Hormones for all women for the rest of their lives' was the catchphrase of the drug companies; HRT went global and became one of the most prescribed treatments for women over the age of 40.

It wasn't until the late 1980s that reports surfaced of breast cancer being linked to the use of HRT. The response was a marketing push that suggested that the benefits of HRT outweighed the risks. In fact, it seemed to the public that the risk of not taking HRT could still be much worse. Without taking hormones, our bones would crumble, we would suffer heart disease or stroke and our quality of life would decrease significantly. Doctors, too, were still advising their patients to keep taking hormones, and our culture does not question the medical fraternity.

## HRT ON TRIAL

In the 1990s pressure mounted for an unbiased judgement on whether HRT was best for women's health. After decades of lobbying, women's health advocacy brought about several large-scale hormone studies investigating the safety of HRT. The news became increasingly unfavourable for the pro-HRT camp.

In 1991, a US-government-funded Women's Health Initiative (WHI) study started to track 161 000 women who were either on a combination of Premarin and Provera, Premarin alone or on a placebo. Although the trial was set to run for 10 years, it had to be called off prematurely due to ethical concerns. Three years before the planned completion of the trial, it had become clear that there was a greater than expected incidence of breast cancer in the HRT group. Not only that, but women in the same group were more likely to suffer from blood clots, which could cause strokes and heart attacks.

This staggering discovery made front-page news across the globe in June 2002. The argument that the benefits of HRT outweighed the risks was proved to be irrevocably flawed. Although it was a triumph of science over marketing, the results left women with a terrible choice to make: take HRT and put themselves at risk of devastating diseases or face the life-altering symptoms of menopause unsupported.

## WHAT NOW?

Since 2002, millions of women have stopped their HRT and concerned practitioners have been exploring the alternatives.

Of course, the pharmaceutical industry is not giving up. It too is looking for alternatives to conventional HRT. Menopausal women make up a demanding and active market, and it's in the industry's interest to keep menopausal women on medication. The drug companies have not been very inventive in their search for a solution, however. The great 'new' hope for menopausal women now seems to be the antidepressant. We have come full circle – women were put on antidepressants and sedatives in the 1960s, and now, 50 years later, these drugs are being touted as our best option. And this is what we call progress!

This is where this book comes in. Our aim is to help you understand what your body is going through during menopause and other times of hormonal disarray. Women have become fearful of their own bodies, and it is vital that we all understand our hormones: what they do and why we need them. Women should know, too, that they have a choice when it comes to conventional HRT and that there is a safe alternative. This book was written to help women make an informed decision and to help them discuss these matters with their doctor without feeling intimidated. It's our hope that it will give each woman the knowledge and confidence she needs to make the right choice for herself.

# 2
# all about bio-identical hormone therapy

## THE TRUTH ABOUT BIO-IDENTICAL HORMONES

There's a lot of contradictory information about bio-identical hormones out there. Many concerns – understandably – centre on the efficacy and safety of these hormones. I've heard medical practitioners say everything from 'bio-identicals are just placebos' to 'I've never heard of them so they can't be any good'. Of course people feel uncertain or insecure about undertaking a treatment that isn't supported by their GP, but this is a conflict that often arises in complementary medicine. Here I'll do my utmost to lay out the facts – the pros and the cons – about using bio-identical hormones.

To my mind the debate must be put in context – we must compare natural bio-identical hormones with synthetic hormones and assess their differences and similarities. We use 'bio-identical' to describe hormones that are chemically identical to our own. Admittedly the term 'natural' is overused – and in some cases abused – when it comes to describing medical treatments. In the case of bio-identical hormones I use it to signify that the hormones both conform to nature and occur naturally. They are produced in our body and are therefore naturally occurring substances. Bio-identical hormones are the same as naturally occurring hormones. Synthetic hormones are manmade drugs that act as hormones. This is their major difference: one is a drug and like all drugs has a defined side-effect profile, the other is a hormone. Hormones are chemical substances that control the body's metabolic processes. They are not drugs.

## THE DISCOVERY OF HORMONES

The term 'hormone' was first used in 1896 by the Viennese gynaecologist Emil Knauer, who wrote of the existence of some 'mysterious chemicals which controlled a variety of metabolic processes in the body'. He named these chemicals 'hormones', from the Greek word *hormao*, to 'stir up' or 'incite'. A few years earlier, in 1889, Dr Edouard Brown-Séquard had announced that he was 'rejuvenated' after injecting himself with a mixture of guinea pig and dog testicle extracts. This led to a short-lived spell of interest into the research of sex-gland extracts as a possible source for a 'fountain of youth'.

In 1928, scientists at the University of Rochester in New York identified the ovarian hormone progesterone and its crucial role in preparing the uterus for pregnancy. The following year, the sex hormone oestrogen was isolated and identified by Drs Edward Doisy and Edgar Allen at Washington University in St Louis. Together they established the existence of oestrogen and described its effects.

Once scientists had isolated progesterone and oestrogen and determined their chemical structure, they explored their possible therapeutic effects, hoping that hormone treatments would be effective for gynaecological disorders. Both scientists and drug manufacturers saw hormone research as having the potential to cure a wide range of medical conditions.

In 1933, Ayerst Labs marketed a product it made from the urine of pregnant women and called Emmenin. This was the first oral oestrogen-replacement product, but due to high production costs and problems with taste and odour, Ayerst Labs began research almost immediately into a new source of oestrogen. They turned to stallions, which were known to have the most potent form of oestrogen in their urine, but they were too wild and frequently kicked over the collection buckets. Pregnant mares proved to be a more placid and much better source. Their urine was at least two and a half times as potent as human urine! Ayerst named the product Premarin, which was a contraction of the drug's description: PREgnant MAres' uRINe.

At the same time, Schering in Germany was working on formulations for the treatment of menopausal symptoms. Schering, which also used human pregnancy urine as the raw material for a product it called Progynon, sought a different source. Extracting progesterone from animal sources was time-consuming and prohibitively expensive (US$80–1000 per gram), both major obstacles in manufacturing it for the public. In 1938, scientists at Schering synthesised ethinylestradiol, the most popular form of oestrogen used in birth control pills to this very day.

As we have seen, it was Russell Marker who discovered a way to extract progesterone from plants. His method, now known as the Marker degradation process, is used by all pharmaceutical companies in the manufacture of bio-identical and synthetic hormones. Marker's breakthrough was to isolate progesterone from plants such as yam or soya, which then enabled oestrogens and testosterone to be produced from the one source.

Progesterone could not be used orally until 1951, when Syntax Laboratories in Mexico discovered norenthindrone, the first orally active synthetic progesterone. It became the other main ingredient in the first oral contraceptive and is still used today in half of all oral contraceptive pills.

## BIO-IDENTICALS AND BRAND NAMES

I've heard criticism from some medical professionals that bio-identical hormones are 'unproven' and 'unsafe'. This is a fallacy. Some forms of bio-identical hormones are produced and manufactured by major pharmaceutical companies. These preparations are readily available under their proprietary names: Crinone and Utrogest, for example, are bio-identical progesterone gels prescribed to treat infertility. In fact, they are the only progesterone products approved by the US Food and Drug Administration for treating infertility and for use during pregnancy. Cyclogest, a progesterone suppository, is prescribed for premenstrual stress; Gestone, a progesterone injection, is prescribed for recurrent miscarriages; and Utrogestan, a progesterone capsule or vaginal suppository, is prescribed for recurrent miscarriages and is added to oestrogen in an HRT regime.

Similarly, there are several bio-identical oestradiol and oestriol products on the market: Sandrena and Oestrogel are oestradiol hormones available as topical gels; Elleste-Solo is an oestradiol tablet; and Estraderm is an oestradiol patch. Hormonin is a combination of oestradiol, oestriol and oestrone in one tablet. Vagifem is an oestradiol vaginal tablet and Ovestin is an oestriol cream prescribed for vaginal dryness.

Bio-identical testosterone is also available – in different forms for women and men – as Testosterone Implants, gels (Testogel) and patches (Intrinsa).

All of these products are bio-identical hormones manufactured by major pharmaceutical companies and sold under their brand names. They have all undergone strict trials and testing in order to be approved by the Australian Therapeutic Goods Administration (TGA) or the US Food and Drug Administration (FDA) and the Medicines and Healthcare products Regulatory Agency (MHRA) in the UK. Bio-identical hormones – oestradiol, oestriol, progesterone and testosterone – have been tested, approved and registered.

The difference between these pharmacological bio-identical hormones and the ones I recommend is that the latter are not manufactured in a uniform way; they are individually formulated by a prescribing doctor and made up by a pharmacist. Only compounding pharmacies have a licence to compound (make up) preparations from a doctor's prescription, so it is very important to work with a reputable accredited compounding pharmacist who complies with rigorous compounding standards under close pharmacist supervision, and who works closely with both doctor and patient to ensure consistency of the compounded product and reduce any risk associated with inaccurate compounding or dosage instructions.

The hormones sold by pharmaceutical companies under their brand names are the same as those used by a pharmacist to create compounded formulations. Many doctors are not even aware of this. They may rubbish natural progesterone cream but condone and prescribe the use of Utrogest vaginal suppositories for fertility treatment.

## SAFETY CONCERNS

The medical fraternity has also denounced bio-identical hormones by saying that if they have the same effects as conventional HRT, then they may have the same risks and dangers.

Conventional HRT, however, is a combination of *synthetic* oestrogens, such as Premarin, Delestrogen and ethinylestradiol; and progestins (synthetic progesterones), such as norethisterone, medroxy-progesterone acetate or dydrogesterone. None of these has the same molecular structure as its bio-identical counterparts. It therefore does not necessarily follow that they have the same side effects.

Some studies into the efficacy and side-effect profile of such bio-identical hormones as oestradiol and progesterone have been carried out. One paper, published in the *Annals of the New York Academy of Sciences* in 2005, compiled observations and results from 23 years of clinical and laboratory practice and many papers concur that bio-identical hormones are safe but as effective as conventional HRT.

Oestrogen, progesterone and testosterone administered in physiological amounts do not have side effects. It is the lack or excess of one or all hormones that can cause problems or unwanted side effects. Too much progesterone can cause fatigue, too little can cause anxiety; too much oestrogen can cause bleeding, too little can cause insomnia or dry skin; too much testosterone can cause acne or aggressive behaviour, too little can cause joint pain or lack of confidence. Everyone will react differently to the effects of these hormones and it is for this reason that doctors need to treat each patient with an individual approach and solution.

## PROTECTION AGAINST OSTEOPOROSIS AND UTERINE CANCER

The medical fraternity has also argued that bio-identical hormones don't protect us from osteoporosis or uterine cancer in the same ways as does conventional HRT. They say that women will start to lose bone density as they approach menopause and their ovaries cease producing oestrogen, progesterone and testosterone.

In the last 15 years of prescribing bio-identical hormones I have witnessed significant improvements in the bone density of most of my patients who have either osteopaenia (thin bones) or osteoporosis (brittle bones). Various studies have proven that progesterone is a bone-building hormone. Good nutrition, weight-bearing exercise and treatment with bio-identical hormones have all been shown to contribute to bone health and bone strength.

There is also evidence from the American Association for Cancer Research that bio-identical hormones help protect the uterus lining from becoming too thick. This phenomenon, which we call endometrial hyperplasia, can occur if you take too much oestrogen and can be a precursor to cancer of the womb.

## BUT DO THEY WORK?

Lastly, the medical establishment has called into question the efficacy of bio-identical hormones – some doctors simply contend that they don't work. Apart from trials that clearly refute these claims, there are the case studies throughout this book. In my 15 years of prescribing bio-identical hormones, I have seen first-hand, time after time, how these treatments have helped my patients. Bio-identical hormones *do* work.

As an informed patient, you need to be armed with this type of information when you visit your GP. At times he or she may not have the knowledge you have. If you have a good relationship with your doctor and there is mutual respect, then you can work as a team for your benefit. Never forget that *you* employ your doctor to advise and treat you, and that you have a legitimate say in the form this treatment takes.

## TWO POWERFUL EXAMPLES

Before we get to the nitty-gritty of the role each major hormone plays in our body, let's take a look at how bio-identical hormone therapy has turned the lives of the following two women around. Treating them provided me with two of the most satisfying and positive experiences I have had as a doctor.

# Petra's story

## PERI-MENOPAUSAL BUT STILL HOPING FOR A BABY

**The Hormone Doctor:** Petra first came to see me when she was 47 years old. She was experiencing some hot flushes, her periods had become irregular and she wanted to understand what was happening. Petra had married at the age of 42, and she and her husband desperately wanted to have a baby.

Petra was extremely attractive, tall and slim, and looked more like 37 than 47. Her blood tests indicated a high level of follicle-stimulating hormone (FSH), very low oestradiol levels and no detectable progesterone. Petra's results showed that she was peri-menopausal; that is, she was around the time of menopause (*peri* means 'surrounding'). Her irregular periods were most likely anovulatory (without ovulation), as she was not producing enough progesterone to bring about the release of an egg from her ovaries.

I decided to put Petra on a course of bio-identical hormones to balance her peri-menopausal state, prescribing her a low-dose combination of all three oestrogens (oestradiol, oestrone and oestriol) with progesterone. I wanted to mimic the body's natural levels as closely as possible and maintain the hormone balance, topping up what Petra was missing. This brought on Petra's regular periods again.

Petra hoped that she might still ovulate and fall pregnant. I did not discourage the idea of Petra becoming pregnant, but I recognised how unlikely this outcome was. Petra did not come to me for fertility treatment as such, but to assess her hormonal state and to treat her accordingly to help her maintain a cycle. She wanted to minimise all possible effects of low ovarian hormones, such as a dry vagina, dry skin, low energy levels, mood swings, headaches and so on.

After about a year of treatment, Petra's periods stopped completely. Her ovaries ceased to function and tests showed she was no longer producing sufficient amounts of oestradiol, progesterone or testosterone. Petra was menopausal. She continued her bio-hormone replacement treatment, which I adjusted in line with her latest blood tests. Petra had no menopausal symptoms, no hot flushes, no insomnia, no mood swings and said she felt well and energetic.

Petra then started investigating the possibilities of IVF with a donor egg and her husband's sperm. At this time she was 49 years old – by definition post-menopausal and therefore in Australia considered too old for this treatment. Petra could not find an Australian IVF centre that would support her mission to have a baby. I continued to see and treat Petra and admired her tenacity, but at no time did I believe that she would be successful in her quest.

At an appointment two years later, she burst in to my office, excited because she had found a Russian IVF centre willing to take her on as a patient. The egg donor would be a young Russian woman who had similar features to Petra. This time I nearly rolled my eyes in disbelief: I had prejudices about Russia's medical system and, after all, Petra was nearly 52! I didn't say anything, however. I just handed over her latest prescription and wished her well.

About 18 months later I saw Petra again in my waiting room, looking as beautiful and calm as ever. When I called her into my office, she sat down and, smiling, took something out of her handbag. It was a photo of twin babies, a boy and a girl. I was speechless. Petra was 54 and had four-month-old twins.

She told me what had happened. She didn't end up going to Russia but had gone to a South African fertility clinic instead. There, embryos created from the eggs of a young South African student and Petra's husband's sperm were implanted in Petra's womb. One implantation failed, but the second was successful. When she was six weeks pregnant, she flew back to Sydney and continued a normal pregnancy under the close supervision of her obstetrician. Petra bore healthy twins by caesarean section shortly before she turned 54. Although she never went public, Petra is probably the oldest woman in Australia to have borne twins.

How was this possible? Petra had been post-menopausal for at least five years, but her bio-identical hormone treatment had helped her uterus to remain healthy: it had a good blood supply and did not atrophy as expected in a post-menopausal woman. Biologically, Petra was 10 years younger than her actual age, but also mentally and emotionally she always remained confident that she could be a mother. She never experienced menopausal symptoms: hot flushes, sleepless nights, terrible mood swings or periods of anxiety or depression. Petra never lost her energy or vitality.

I find this story so inspiring because Petra never gave up. She had a better chance of winning the lottery than getting pregnant, but she believed in herself and had the confidence to carry her dream through to fruition. This would never have happened without her stubbornness or persistence, but I believe that bio-identical hormones played their role too.

**The Nutritionist:** This is an extraordinary story, but fertility can concern women far younger than Petra. Not everyone needs hormone supplementation to support a successful, healthy pregnancy, but good nutrition is vital for both the mother and the developing foetus. Petra's diet and lifestyle were without fault, but sadly too many women (and men) do not look after their health when planning a family.

I always recommend that would-be mothers keep as much of their diet as organic as possible – no developing baby needs pesticide residues. Fabulous fertility foods include all animal proteins containing zinc (eggs, poultry, lean red meat, fish), which is vital for physical growth as well as the development of the neurological and immune systems. Also good for those trying to conceive are all whole grains, which contain the full range of B-group vitamins, as well as nuts and seeds, which are required for the growth of the brain and nervous system.

Whole grains, seeds and nuts are also excellent for providing ongoing energy for the mother and developing baby. Fresh-water and deep-sea fish, nuts, seeds and their oils all provide a wonderful range of omega-3, -6 and -9 fatty acids, which help to create every cell in the body.

Throughout this book I will recommend 'megafoods' for each section – these are the foods that you should definitely add to your weekly shopping list. Regularly eating these foods will guarantee that you're getting the nutrients you need to help combat your particular symptoms.

## Fertility megafoods

- pomegranate, kiwifruit and all berries (fresh or frozen because the vitamin status of frozen berries is the same as fresh)
- wild salmon, sardines in their own oil, monkfish (try to ensure that your fish has had minimum exposure to pollutants)
- barley, buckwheat, quinoa, oats
- watercress, rocket, curly kale, spinach, Savoy cabbage, seaweeds, pumpkin, squash, peppers and cucumber (cucumber is rich in potassium, which helps to keep down blood pressure and fluid retention during pregnancy)
- almonds, flaxseed, pumpkin and sunflower seeds
- best quality steak or lean lamb cutlets

In addition to these fresh foods, I recommend taking specific nutrient supplements for at least six months before and then throughout your pregnancy. Many combinations have been formulated for pre-conception and pregnancy care, but they should always include the following.

| Supplement | Daily dosage | Good for ... |
| --- | --- | --- |
| B-complex vitamins | At least 50 milligrams each | Growth and development |
| Thiamin (B1) | 25 milligrams | Nervous system |
| Riboflavin (B2) | 25 milligrams | Metabolism of fats and carbohydrates |
| Niacin (B3) | 25 milligrams | Cognitive function and mood |
| Pantothenic acid (B5) | 25 milligrams | Balances stress hormones, regulates protein and carbohydrate metabolism |
| Vitamin B6 | 25 milligrams | Neurological and brain function; protein metabolism |
| Vitamin B12 | 1000 IUs | Neurological function and protein metabolism |
| Vitamin C | At least 500 milligrams | Skin and all internal tissue development |
| Vitamin D | 600 IUs | Bones, ligaments and teeth |
| Vitamin E | 50 milligrams | Skin; also an antioxidant |
| Beta-carotene | 50 milligrams | Immunity and the skin |
| Calcium | 200 milligrams | Bone and ligament development |
| Magnesium | 400 milligrams | Cardiovascular system and carbohydrate metabolism |
| Iron ascorbate | 50 milligrams | Blood supply |
| Folic acid | 400 micrograms | Neurological development |
| Zinc citrate | 50 milligrams | Immunity |
| Selenium | 50 micrograms | Immunity and the thyroid |
| Copper | 1 milligram | Metabolism; also has antioxidant properties |
| L-arginine | 100 milligrams | Men: development of healthy sperm |
| N-acetylcholine | 50 milligrams | Digestive tract function |
| Iodine | 140 micrograms | Metabolism, thyroid and growth |

Staying well hydrated is a must, but never drink tap water – it may contain high levels of chlorine, which can be toxic to a developing foetus. To make still bottled water more interesting, try adding some fresh mint leaves, sliced cucumber or pomegranate seeds.

It is important to take care with herbs during pregnancy, as some can be contraindicated, such as raspberry leaf, which can cause contractions. You can use the following herbs safely, fresh, in your cooking, or in delicious herbal teas: peppermint, thyme, basil, fennel, dill and chamomile.

Remember to eat regularly – this will keep your energy levels up and help prevent morning sickness. While ginger is a miracle in itself for nausea, large amounts can be too stimulating, causing palpitations or premature contractions. A thumbnail-long sliver of fresh root ginger or 2 flat teaspoons of powdered ginger in a large cup of hot water is enough each day.

## Tessa's story

### TURNER SYNDROME

**The Hormone Doctor:** Tessa's parents called me a week before my first appointment with her, to 'check me out' to see whether I was the right choice to help their 21-year-old daughter. They informed me that Tessa had been born with Turner Syndrome. This is a chromosomal aberration in women that results in shortness of stature and a short neck. Women with Turner Syndrome may be born with ovaries that never function and a uterus that remains infantile in size and function; these women are infertile and their ovaries are too immature to produce any sex hormones. Maturation of their breasts and sex organs does not take place, and women who have Turner Syndrome lack many of the feminine features we take for granted.

Tessa was initially reluctant to see me, as she had been traumatised by the way some of her doctors and specialists had categorised her. She said she didn't feel 'normal', and that she felt more like a 'freak' than the intelligent young woman she really was.

Tessa was concerned that she would never get her period or develop as a woman. She had been told that she could go onto the pill as a replacement for her own non-functioning ovaries, which would give her a 'normal' period. Tessa's parents, who had researched the possible benefits and side effects of being on synthetic hormones for a whole lifespan, were convinced that there must be a better way and decided to contact me after they had read about me in a women's magazine.

Tessa arrived for the consultation with both her mother and father. Tessa was small and neat, had slightly coarse facial features and undeveloped breasts, but she did not recognisably have Turner Syndrome. Although apprehensive, she was very articulate and stated her position, how she felt and what her concerns were. She was obviously very bright and outspoken. She took control of her situation, as she said that she had felt humiliated by one of her past specialists. This was not to happen again and that was why I had been interrogated before our first meeting.

We discussed her syndrome and what her options were regarding her hormonal treatment. She had brought her ultrasound scans with her – their accompanying report described an 'infantile' uterus and that 'no ovaries could be identified'. She had neither functioning ovaries that could produce follicles for ovulation nor hormones. Sadly, the syndrome meant that Tessa had an increased risk of osteoporosis and would age at an accelerated rate, as she would not enjoy any of the benefits that hormones give the skin, bones, brain and heart. Tessa was reluctant to take anything artificial, but she was also sceptical about the natural, 'normal' bio-identical hormones she had read about.

I explained to the family how easy, safe and uncomplicated treatment with bio-identicals would be. Furthermore, I explained how the hormones would work and that, under their influence, Tessa's ovaries, uterus and genital area would mature. I requested blood tests to confirm her hormonal status. I could later compare these with any blood tests taken after treatment had begun. I also felt that seeing the changes would make Tessa and her family more confident.

I put Tessa on a combination of oestradiol and progesterone in a cream form that she was to apply twice daily. She responded to the treatment practically immediately, and excitedly rang me up after three weeks exclaiming that she had noticed a slight vaginal discharge. What for us may be cumbersome and irritating made Tessa feel like a 'normal woman'. After six months we repeated her pelvic ultrasound and her uterus was described as 'small and normal'. No more references to it as 'infantile'.

There were other developments, too. Tessa's moods had changed. She became more content and self-confident. She had needed to buy a bra for her newly developed small breasts. She was becoming more feminine. There was great excitement when she had her first period.

When this started happening, I asked Tessa to apply the hormones in a cyclical manner, mimicking a monthly cycle. Tessa and her parents were thrilled with the results. Tessa is not only happy but also very pretty now. Her facial features have softened and she feels like a woman – she feels normal. This has not only changed her life, but also that of her parents. They can see how she has developed and has overcome her depression regarding her genetic condition. She is a happy young woman who is leading a normal life, and this has lifted a load from everyone's shoulders. Replacing Tessa's missing hormones with natural bio-identical hormones has assured her and her family a normal life.

# 3

# all about oestrogen

## THE MOST ANCIENT OF ALL HORMONES

Did you know that oestrogen is the most ancient of all hormones? Scientists have found traces of it in matter that is more than 650 million years old!

Well, it can't be such a bad thing if it has been around since time began. In fact, oestrogen is very powerful and evolution has given it to women. Yes, men have a little bit too, but they don't like to admit it. Oestrogen is the hormone that makes women feel, look and behave like women. It shapes our emotions and our bodies.

Oestrogen is in fact a name given to a group of female hormones that are produced in our ovaries during childhood, puberty and our fertile years until menopause. These hormones are known as oestradiol, which is very potent; oestrone, which is less powerful; and oestriol, which is weak and very safe and which we have in abundance, particularly during pregnancy, when the embryo is literally bathed in it.

Oestrogens are the hormones that transform a girl into a woman. They are the essence of feminine energy and vitality. They make us feel feminine and sexy – they shape our breasts and hips, they help to control menstruation and pregnancy, and they give a sparkle to our eyes. But along with bestowing uniquely female attributes, oestrogens perform many other vital tasks. They regulate body temperature, help you sleep deeply, support the collagen in your skin, help maintain your memory, concentration and bone density, and help keep your moods positive. Oestrogens protect you from cardiovascular disease and assist in the formation of neurotransmitters such as serotonin, which decreases depression, irritability and anxiety. This is one of the reasons why some women suddenly develop anxiety and panic attacks when they head towards or hit menopause and their body's production of oestrogens decreases. So many of my patients complain that they have become very anxious and worry about nothing. Some have such severe panic attacks that they no longer want to drive over bridges or through tunnels or even go out on their own.

Since oestrogens are so good for us, wouldn't it be wonderful if our ovaries maintained their function throughout our lifetime? Then we wouldn't have to undergo oestrogen-withdrawal symptoms when we reach menopause.

## BIO-IDENTICAL VERSUS SYNTHETIC OESTROGENS

Now please bear with me while I explain the difference between bio-identical oestrogens, which *replicate* our own hormones, and therefore can be used to replace our hormones, and the synthetic ones, which *mimic* the actions of our hormones, and can only be considered as a substitute and not replacement therapy.

Bio-identical hormones are an exact copy of the hormones we produce. Synthetic hormones, on the other hand, are not the same as they have neither the same molecular structure nor efficacy. Synthetic hormones may be, at times, more potent than our own and therefore may have detrimental or unwanted side effects. These synthetic hormones are often prescribed in conventional HRT therapy.

# PREMARIN IS NOT OESTROGEN!

Premarin is the most common 'oestrogenic' compound prescribed to menopausal women throughout the world. But where does it come from and how does it differ from our own hormones?

Premarin comes from PREgnant MAres' uRINe. Yes, that's right, women are swallowing horses' hormones, which are chemically different from their own. Look at these diagrams of the molecular structures of Premarin and oestradiol – you don't need a PhD in chemistry to see how different they are.

*Oestradiol*

*Premarin*

Premarin differs from our oestrogens not only in its molecular (chemical) structure but also in its potency – clearly we do not have the enzymes (that horses do) to metabolise or break down equilin (horses' oestrogen). Therefore the effects of Premarin are not only much more potent than those of our own oestrogens, but we also tend to accumulate it for longer periods of time, leading to the side effects we have all heard about – if not experienced – and want to avoid.

It is no coincidence that one of the major problems for women who are put on conventional HRT (Premarin and Provera) is weight gain. They complain of increased breast size and bloating, and that they no longer fit into their clothes and have to buy a new wardrobe at least two sizes larger. These very strong and potent hormones are meant for horses and not women.

You may now ask, 'Well, why are we being prescribed Premarin and not bio-identical oestrogens?' The answer is very simple. Premarin could be patented and therefore owned by the pharmaceutical company that developed it. Oestrogens, however, are substances that already occur in nature, and what already exists in nature cannot, in itself, be patented. There is little profit to be made for a pharmaceutical company in researching and marketing a naturally existing substance that another company could quickly copy and profit from (there are, however, a small number of exceptions to this – see page 36). There is a strong incentive for pharmaceutical companies to develop synthetic, patent-able products. And, after considerable expense developing it, researching it and marketing it, they do not want any other company to profit from their hard work.

Here's the story of one of my patients who was prescribed Premarin after a total hysterectomy.

## *Caroline's story*

### ALLERGIC REACTION TO PREMARIN: 'EVERY STEP AN EFFORT'

**The Hormone Doctor:** Caroline is 48 years old and had a total hysterectomy (removal of the uterus and both ovaries) at the age of 43. Caroline had what we call a surgical menopause because her ovaries were removed at the same time as her uterus and from one day to the next she became oestrogen-, progesterone- and testosterone-depleted. She was put on Premarin immediately after her operation to counteract hormone-withdrawal symptoms such as hot flushes and insomnia. Her doctors did not even consider replacing her progesterone and testosterone!

Shortly after the operation Caroline developed very severe asthma and had to be put on steroid medication. She gained weight and became quite depressed. She stayed on Premarin for the next three years. In the last two years before she visited me, her doctor had changed her prescription, giving her a six-monthly oestrogen implant instead of the Premarin.

Caroline was a very pleasant and friendly woman with a beautiful smile, but she seemed totally exhausted and was not coping with her professional and family life. She seemed very despondent. Caroline said she felt 'as if I'm walking through mud and every step is an effort'.

While I was taking her history, Caroline told me that she had had a total hysterectomy because of dysfunctional uterine bleeding. She needed to have her uterus taken out because she was bleeding very heavily, had clots and flooding and was anaemic. I asked her why she had also had her ovaries removed. At the time of the operation she had been casually advised that her ovaries could remain in if they were not diseased but that if they were removed she would never have to worry about getting ovarian cancer. This was all the advice and explanation she was given, and she agreed to their removal.

But did she have to have her ovaries removed? I always ask my patients to come armed with as much medical information as possible, such as past blood tests, X-rays and reports from specialists. Caroline had a copy of her surgical report, which said, 'both left and right ovaries appeared normal'. And yet they were removed! I read this with such shame. How could any surgeon remove such important organs, especially from a relatively young woman when there was nothing wrong with them? Ovaries are so vital for producing hormones that maintain healthy bone, tissue, brain function, energy, mood and so much more.

Well, this is when all the trouble started for Caroline. While she took 0.625 milligrams of Premarin daily for the next three years, she put on about 10 kilograms and developed severe asthma. For the first time in her life her asthma was so bad that she was put on steroid medication to control it. Although she didn't experience hot flushes, she was struggling with a lack of energy and laboured breathing. Her asthma attacks were so bad that she had been hospitalised twice.

Caroline then had allergy testing and discovered she was allergic to horse hair and horse dust mites. Poor Caroline – she had been given horses' hormone to swallow for three years! Thank goodness that an enlightened doctor ordered allergy testing for her.

Caroline stopped taking Premarin and was given an oestrogen implant instead. Although her asthma improved dramatically, her energy levels and moods did not. When Caroline arrived at her first consultation with me, she said, 'I feel like a shell of a person . . . the lights are on but no one's home.' She felt like life was a constant struggle; she could neither experience joy nor look forward to the future.

Caroline's blood tests confirmed what I had suspected: she had no testosterone, no progesterone and very low levels of DHEA-S (a hormone precursor). She had oestradiol in sufficient amounts but she may have needed more.

Why is it common practice for doctors to replace only oestrogen when the ovaries are removed? Ovaries also produce testosterone and progesterone, and we need these hormones for our confidence, libido, moods, vitality, bones and for many more reasons. Nature intended us to have all of these hormones. With bio-identical hormone replacement (and in this case it was a matter of 'replacement' rather than 'supplementation', because there were no more ovaries to produce these vital hormones), we try to copy what nature planned for us with hormones identical to those that nature made for us.

I prescribed Caroline a lozenge that dissolves in the mouth and releases the hormones directly into the bloodstream through the mucus membranes. I gave her a combination of oestradiol (as her most recent implant had run out) and progesterone, which is a calming hormone, to help with her anxiety and her feeling of being overwhelmed by life. I also gave her a very small amount of testosterone, to give her a feeling of vitality and confidence. The testosterone would also be beneficial for her bones.

I asked Caroline to see me in six weeks and report back on how she was feeling. Often at these follow-up appointments it is necessary to do some fine-tuning of the prescribed dosages in response to my patients' needs. Everyone is different and requires an individual approach to their treatment, even though their symptoms may be similar.

At this second appointment, Caroline was smiling. She had lost some weight, she looked and felt relieved, and her eyes were sparkling. She said that she had 'found her old self' again. Her libido and energy had improved (although there was still room for more improvement) and she was much more optimistic about her future. She could not believe the difference taking the bio-identical hormones had made. She felt like a 'whole woman again'; whole because she had her hormones back and could function once more.

## Leave healthy ovaries alone

So why is Caroline's story so significant? First of all, Caroline's ovaries were removed even though there was nothing wrong with them. In my opinion this is a medical misdemeanour. In my practice I have seen so many patients whose ovaries (and uterus) have been removed unnecessarily. Unfortunately, some women have very strong negative emotional reactions to what has happened to them. Anger, depression and a sense of mourning are just some of the emotions women may experience after having a hysterectomy (removal of the uterus) or total hysterectomy (removal of the uterus and ovaries). Because of this surgical intervention, women are suddenly confronted with the end of a very significant episode in their lives. Their fertile years are over; for some this can be synonymous with a loss of their femininity, attractiveness and sense of worth. (Of course, these are also emotions that many women experience when they approach or reach menopause more gradually.) The unnecessary removal of the uterus and/or ovaries is not only detrimental to health but also to emotional wellbeing.

The fear of the possibility of ovarian cancer was instilled into Caroline, but should we be driven by fear? She thought, 'Okay, let them go. One less thing to worry about.' Does this mean that all women beyond their fertile age should have their ovaries removed to prevent cancer? Certainly not! Taking responsibility for our health is the best way: a better lifestyle, good nutrition, stress management, exercise and a healthy curiosity about our environment will help us take control of our life and health.

The major problem in Caroline's case was that she was given a hormone drug, Premarin, that was foreign to her body, which reacted to it as such. She was allergic to it and developed such severe asthma that she nearly succumbed to it twice. But the other problem was that she was prescribed neither progesterone nor testosterone, both of which her ovaries had been producing until they were removed. Women are naturally meant to benefit not only from oestrogen but also progesterone and testosterone – we need them all.

There is a belief in the medical profession that if a woman has had her uterus removed, she no longer needs progesterone. This attitude comes from the early days of ERT (oestrogen replacement therapy). All women were given Premarin for their menopausal symptoms in the 1970s until the medical fraternity discovered that this was the cause of uterine cancer in women taking Premarin alone. This 'unopposed oestrogen therapy' – when oestrogen is prescribed without the balancing effect of progesterone – allowed the lining of the uterus to grow (endometrial hyperplasia) under the influence of oestrogen. To counteract these effects, a progestin, a synthetic progesterone (usually the drug Provera), was added to the ERT regime for women who still had a uterus – but it was omitted for women whose uterus had been removed.

Our body produces progesterone not only for pregnancy but also to counteract the growth effects of oestrogen in all tissues. One of its many benefits is its effect on the lining of the uterus, but it also has a protective effect in the breasts and on bone-building. If oestrogen is not finely balanced with progesterone, fibroids, heavy bleeding, endometriosis and breast cysts may develop, and we will not have the best protection for our bones. Our ovarian hormones never work alone – they harmonise with each other and can also be converted into each other as the body requires. So when our hormones are out of tune, we feel out of whack.

Had Caroline received bio-identical oestrogens, progesterone and testosterone from the very beginning, she would never have suffered the adverse side effects. Her life would have remained on track as if she still had her ovaries, which were programmed to produce hormones for another 10 years until her likely menopause.

Common sense dictates that if nature intended us to profit from all the hormones we produce, then we should try to balance or replace them to reflect as closely as possible what would occur naturally. Bio-identical hormones are essential for women (and men) who need their own hormones balanced or replaced, but they can only be prescribed on a one-on-one basis. You are unique, your endocrine system is as unique as your fingerprint, and this is how you need to be treated to get an optimal response from hormone therapy.

**The Nutritionist:** From a nutritional point of view, Caroline's story is, sadly, one I have heard all too often in my clinic – severe allergic reaction to medications that have been prescribed without due consideration. Caroline knew she had had an allergic reaction to horse hair from a young age, but she didn't make the connection that Premarin would bring about that sort of reaction in her. Nor did anyone with greater medical knowledge draw her attention to the fact that Premarin was derived from horses and that she should have her allergies tested before taking the drug.

As we know, some cases of asthma are caused by allergies, where the inflammatory response makes the immune system go haywire. In such cases, an anti-inflammatory diet can bring significant relief. The important thing, if you are trying to follow an anti-inflammatory diet, is to stick to it completely; half-measures are just as bad as not following the diet at all. If you suffer from debilitating allergic reactions, consider incorporating into your diet the following anti-inflammatory foods, avoiding these pro-inflammatory foods and including the following nutritional supplements.

## Anti-inflammatory foods to stock up on

- flaxseeds and flaxseed oil
- pumpkin seeds, sunflower seeds, and their cold-pressed oils – great to add to salad dressings
- pineapple, raspberries, blackberries, plums, peaches, nectarines and almonds
- garlic and onions
- beetroot, pumpkins and sweet potatoes
- sea vegetables – for example, nori seaweed used in sushi
- avocados
- oily fish

## Pro-inflammatory foods to avoid

- nightshades (from the Solanaceae family of plants) – these vegetables and spices are known to be primary irritants in rheumatoid arthritis, as they cause an inflammatory response in the joints; avoid eggplant (aubergines), paprika, chilli, capsicum (bell peppers), potatoes, zucchini (courgettes), tomatoes and tobacco (time to quit if you haven't already)
- cow's dairy produce – all of it; choose goat's, rice or soy milk instead
- wheat and all its derivatives (however delicious they may be) – biscuits, cakes, crackers, croissants, bagels, cereals and wheat-based breads
- some nuts – allergy testing is vital here to determine if you have any allergies
- eggs – these sit at number five on the list of the most common food intolerances, so it's definitely worth being tested

- red meat – highly pro-inflammatory for those who have a tendency for food allergies; as they say, 'One man's meat is another man's poison.'

---

*Did you know . . . ?*

If you have an allergy to peanuts, you shouldn't touch sesame seeds (or tahini, or even hummus made with tahini), as they come from the same plant family.

---

**The five most common food intolerances**

1. cow's dairy
2. citrus fruits
3. nuts (especially peanuts), including sesame seeds
4. gluten (found in wheat, rye and barley and, to a lesser extent, in oats)
5. eggs, either the white (albumen) or the yolk

---

## Supportive supplements

Caroline's case is a prime example of when supportive supplements really are of the essence. Choose multivitamins and minerals that include as many of the following supplements as possible, and add those that are found separately, such as omega-3, bromelain and quercetin.

| Supplement | Daily dosage | Good for ... |
| --- | --- | --- |
| Magnesium | 500 milligrams | Helps relax the bronchial passages and aids deeper breathing |
| Calcium | 250 milligrams | Vital for the contraction of smooth muscle tissue – it works in tandem with magnesium |
| Vitamin C (as mixed ascorbates) | 3–5 grams | Lowers histamine levels that cause inflammatory responses such as itching |
| Omega-3 (consisting of DHA and EPA) | 1000 milligrams | Potent anti-inflammatory |
| Vitamin E | 400 micrograms | Reduces inflammation of bronchial tissues |
| Vitamin B3 ('non-flushing niacin') | 25 milligrams | Lowers histamine levels |
| Quercetin | 300 milligrams | Potent anti-inflammatory |
| Bromelain | 150 milligrams | Reduces inflammation in the lungs associated with asthma |
| Methionine | 50 milligrams | Repairs skin tissue – both internal and external (lungs, gut lining, outer skin) |

## Exercise for allergy-sufferers

If you suffer from allergies and in particular asthma, you need to look at doing specific types of exercise – those that encourage deep, slow breathing. Yoga, Pilates and Tai Chi are great examples that also reduce stress, which can exacerbate any inflammatory or allergic condition.

Learning methods of deep relaxation can be hugely beneficial in all situations. The Buteyko method of breathing has undergone several rigorous trials to test its claim to alleviate asthma and other types of breathing difficulties including anxiety.

*Did you know . . . ?*

Uterus is a Latin word meaning 'womb', and *hystericus* is a Greek word meaning 'of the womb'. In centuries past, hysteria was thought to be a neurotic condition specific to women and caused by a dysfunction of the uterus.

## HYSTERECTOMY: TO KEEP OR NOT TO KEEP YOUR UTERUS?

Initially, when we decided to write this book, hysterectomy was not top of the list of our subjects to cover. Hysterectomy is not a symptom – it is an act or result of a certain medical condition, and sometimes an overreaction on the part of a surgeon or gynaecologist. But I have had countless patients who have been totally devastated by the loss of their uterus, so this is a topic that is clearly relevant to many women. Women who have undergone hysterectomy often go through a phase of bereavement, especially anger, desperation and depression. One of my patients explained: 'It's like coming to terms with death.'

Hysterectomy is the operative removal of the uterus and total hysterectomy is the removal of the uterus, fallopian tubes and ovaries. Hysterectomy is probably one of the most frequently performed operations in the Western world – and the most unnecessary. I am sure that many readers will either have had a hysterectomy or had one recommended for treatment of fibroids or bleeding irregularities. Certainly many of us have friends who have had a hysterectomy.

How many of us have heard the argument 'You've had your family and don't need a uterus any more'? Or 'We should also remove your ovaries to avoid problems in the future'? Or 'If you have your uterus removed, you no longer have to worry about having periods'? These are some of the many reasons given for women to have a hysterectomy.

But how many of us have been told about the psychological importance of the uterus, what the uterus and ovaries mean to a woman's psyche and her identity as a woman, why they are immensely important organs, even if she is no longer going to have babies? Who has explained to us the role of the ovaries and the hormones they produce? Most commonly, the advice and information we receive plays on our fears: 'If you have everything removed, then you won't get ovarian, uterine or cervical cancer.' Makes sense maybe, but then we might as well start removing other body parts as well. Try convincing a man to have his prostate removed to avoid getting prostate cancer. After all, cancer of the prostate is the most common form of cancer in men.

Here are three case studies that relate to this important matter. Each of these patents came to me in the same week and I couldn't believe what I was hearing. I thought the medical profession was long past recommending this antiquated solution and, where it was recommended, would at least offer adequate advice for women to make an informed choice.

## Christa's story

### GOING 'MAD' AFTER A HYSTERECTOMY

**The Hormone Doctor:** When Christa arrived in my waiting room, it was immediately obvious that she was very agitated. Christa started telling me her story: how she had had a hysterectomy six weeks before and that she had been feeling 'mad' ever since.

Christa had been diagnosed with a large fibroid, the size of an orange, about 10 weeks earlier. It had begun to press against her bladder and was causing irritation and the need to urinate frequently. To feel safe wherever she went, Christa needed to know that there would be a toilet nearby. She never imagined that the problem could have been caused by a fibroid, and when her doctor discovered it, Christa was told that it should be removed 'to avoid further problems'. Her gynaecologist informed her that she should have a hysterectomy instead of just a fibroidectomy (removal of the fibroid). He recommended this be done using keyhole surgery. He made it sound like an effortless operation, with no abdominal scarring save for three small incision marks on the abdomen. She agreed but insisted that her ovaries remain intact, as she was still menstruating regularly and had no peri-menopausal symptoms although she was already 52.

Three days after the operation, Christa was discharged from hospital, but she developed a fever and strong pain and had to be readmitted as she was bleeding internally. She had to be re-operated on to remove an internal clot and to cauterise the source of the bleed.

Exactly a fortnight after the first operation she said she started feeling 'mad'. She became incredibly anxious, could not sleep, developed severe hot flushes day and night, and could not control her irritability or panic. She tried to mask this from her family, and especially from her husband, who always considered her to be his 'rock'. Christa felt as if she'd gone from being capable and confident in all situations to losing her mind. She was convinced she was going 'mad'. She felt that this had to do with the operation, as everything had been 'normal' until then, but she couldn't understand why.

Christa then began researching on the internet and realised that she could have had a fibroidectomy alone and no hysterectomy. She was unforgiving and angry with herself. She regretted her decision so much that it consumed her thoughts every hour of the day. She was not just angry and devastated; she was almost suicidal.

I explained to Christa that her feelings of 'madness' might have been caused by sudden hormonal withdrawal. It is not uncommon for women who have undergone a hysterectomy to experience an early menopause. The blood supply to the ovaries can become compromised after an operation and many women experience the results of a 'surgical menopause'. Christa could not believe this. No one had informed her of these possible consequences before her operation.

I took her blood tests and my suspicions were confirmed. Christa was appalled when she heard this. It did not comfort her to understand *why* she was feeling so depressed and crazy. Her anger increased, especially against herself for being so ignorant as to allow this to happen to her.

I tried to console her and explained that although this 'surgical menopause' was more than unfortunate, her symptoms could be resolved easily with supplementation of bio-identical hormones. Christa understood the logic and agreed to the treatment, but unfortunately she still left my room feeling sad and angry.

In her follow-up appointments, Christa has reported that she is back to feeling more normal. She can't believe now that she felt as crazy as she did, and has come to terms with being menopausal.

## Bingi's story

### ADVICE TO HAVE A HYSTERECTOMY 'JUST DIDN'T FEEL RIGHT'

**The Hormone Doctor:** Two days after Christa's appointment Bingi came to see me. As I was walking up the stairs into my consulting room, I heard my patient giggling behind me. I asked her why she was laughing and she replied that I might think that she was a loony, as she was coming to see me to get a third opinion. I told her that I would tell her at the end of the consultation if I thought this were the case.

Bingi was a large woman of African origin who was in her mid-50s. She was still menstruating regularly but had been dismayed at her protruding stomach the size of a four-month-old pregnancy and caused by a large fibroid. She had no other symptoms – no heavy bleeding or flooding, no pain, no incontinence and no bowel or bladder symptoms.

She had been advised to have an operation to avoid 'future problems'. She was very well informed and had been considering an embolisation of the fibroid, which would stop the blood supply to the fibroid and eventually cause it to shrink. She had been disappointed, however, with the clinic that had been recommended to her. She then saw a gynaecologist who said she could remove the fibroid and leave the uterus alone. The gynaecologist did, however, inform Bingi that if there were complications during the operation, she would then have to perform a hysterectomy. Bingi agreed but when she went to sign the preoperative consent form, she noticed that she was booked in for a hysterectomy, not a fibroidectomy. Bingi felt betrayed and immediately cancelled the operation. She felt that the gynaecologist had had every intention from the beginning of performing a hysterectomy.

This was when Bingi came to see me. She was concerned about her fibroid growing larger, but she was even more concerned about what she should do about it.

First we went through the pros and cons of a hysterectomy. Bingi had no symptoms that justified an operation with all its concomitant risks such as infection or postoperative bleeding (such as happened in Christa's case – see page 63). Fibroids develop as a result of excess oestrogen, because of oestrogen's growth-related properties. It is not uncommon for fibroids to grow during a woman's peri-menopausal years, as this is when levels of oestrogen and progesterone are out of balance, and there often is not enough progesterone to counteract the effects of oestrogen. We know that fibroids begin to shrink after menopause, when oestrogen levels drop. It is extremely rare for fibroids to become cancerous and so the risk of cancer should not be a consideration in their removal.

At the end of our consultation I gave my professional opinion that Bingi was both sane and wise. She had told me that she 'just didn't feel right' about the prospect of a hysterectomy. Bingi had followed her intuition – one of our best tools as women – and had done her research so she could make an informed and educated choice. Instead of recommending, as many doctors do, synthetic progesterone in the form of Provera or a Mirena IUD (which delivers a slow release of a progestogen into the uterus daily), I prescribed a daily dose of bio-identical progesterone cream, which Bingi could rub onto her skin to be absorbed into the bloodstream. I asked her to return in three months for a review. After all, Bingi was nearing menopause and a change was on its way.

## Denise's story

### FALSE DIAGNOSIS LED TO 'CASTRATION'

**The Hormone Doctor:** Denise came into my room accompanied by her husband. She was 49 years old, small and fragile-looking, and she seemed to be insecure. She reported that her problems had all started six months before.

During a routine examination by her GP, Denise had complained of some intermenstrual bleeding. She was referred to a gynaecologist, who did a PAP smear and took a tissue sample of the lining of the uterus. A week later she received a phone call and was told to come into the hospital the following morning. This, unsurprisingly, caused a sleepless and anxious night.

Denise saw her doctor, who bluntly informed her that she had uterine cancer and had to have everything – uterus, ovaries and fallopian tubes – removed as soon as possible. She was told that after the operation she would not be able to take HRT as the cancer was oestrogen-responsive. There was no further discussion, and a date was made for the operation. Denise left the hospital in a daze. She did not confide in her children so as to avoid distressing them.

The operation was performed three weeks later. On the day of her release from hospital, the surgeon advised her of her good fortune: she did not have cancer. In fact, it was only a thickening of the uterus lining with some atypical cells. Of course, she was delighted to hear that she didn't have cancer, but Denise was shocked. Here she was with an empty abdomen for no reason – she could not understand how something like this could happen to her. She had always been conscious of her health and body. She had always been interested in healthy food and a healthy lifestyle, and she enjoyed looking after her family in this manner.

Six months later, she felt crippled and depressed, her body ached and she was anxiety-ridden. She tried to cope, to pull herself together for the sake of her children and husband. She returned to work, but she was consumed with thoughts of the procedure and what had happened to her. She likened her experience to a 'deadened feeling, a castration'. She missed the 'ebb and flow of her body' she had felt before the operation. One of her major concerns was that she no longer felt like a woman; she felt asexual.

I reassured Denise that all her feelings of femininity would return with bio-identical hormone replacement. I advised her that I would replace all the hormones with a combination of oestradiol, oestriol, progesterone and testosterone. I prescribed this combination in a quantity suited specifically to Denise's constitution.

Since beginning the hormone treatment, Denise's health has improved. She feels more like a woman again and more vital, but she is still traumatised by her experience.

**The Nutritionist:** I have not as yet seen any of these three patients, as hysterectomy cases are usually dealt with purely on a medical level. Having suffered from fibroids in my 30s and 40s, however, I have taken a keen interest in the prevention and reduction of fibroids through nutritional means.

My own gynaecologist suggested I consider a hysterectomy in my early 40s, when it became apparent that I had a recurrent fibroid in my uterus. This was explained to me as 'the only permanent way to get rid of the painful condition'. While I had already come to terms with the idea that I was highly unlikely to have children, I was horrified at this extreme 'no-return' option and declined, stating that I would rather put up with the pain and heavy bleeding.

I left my doctor's office determined to find my own solution. Fortunately, I then met Marion, who prescribed me a progesterone cream to help balance my previously unchallenged levels of oestrogen. I consider myself very lucky to have had this option when many others have not. Along with changes to my diet, Marion's treatment has ensured that the fibroid is now virtually non-existent, even though I am well into peri-menopause. This is a perfect example of bio-identical hormones and nutrition playing an equally important role.

These are not unusual cases, and it is vital that all women are prepared for and informed about hysterectomies. Of course, for some a hysterectomy is necessary and even life-saving. There are cases where women have such dysfunctional bleeding that it encroaches on their daily lives. Some cannot leave the house for fear of flooding; others become severely anaemic, and for them a hysterectomy is the right and proper choice. And there are those for whom the uterus has caused problems and pain all their life, and these women can simply be glad to be rid of it. But we need to think also of those who are not told the full story, or who are not given a real choice in the matter.

The medical profession seems to underestimate the psychological importance of the uterus. More care and empathy needs to be used when a woman is faced with losing the symbol of her womanhood.

## Fibroid-aggravating foods to avoid

The following foods are known to aggravate or increase the production of oestrogen in the liver. As fibroids occur as a result of excess or unopposed oestrogen circulating in the body, it is advisable to cut back, or cut out altogether, those foods that could increase the amount of oestrogen produced.

- alcohol
- caffeine (particularly instant coffee)
- cow's dairy products
- milk chocolates
- sugar

## Fibroid megafoods

Foods that support the liver are important when it comes to fibroids, as the liver is the major organ of detoxification and the place where oestrogens are broken down. It is vital that the liver functions optimally to ensure that this oestrogen metabolism is not compromised. Phyto-hormone foods are also vital in preserving the balance of oestrogen and progesterone. Make sure that you consume a selection of these foods on a regular basis.

- asparagus and artichokes (liver-supportive and kidney-cleansing)
- garlic, onions, spring onions and eggs (sulphur-rich foods that support the liver)
- apples and pears (pectin helps to remove toxins from the gut, preventing re-absorption of excess oestrogen)
- soy products – milk, tofu, tempeh and fresh miso soup (phyto-hormone foods)
- pulses and lentils, chickpeas and hummus (more wonderful phyto-hormone foods)
- fennel, chicory, celery, endive and radicchio lettuce (phyto-hormone vegetables)

# WHEN 'CRAZY LADY SYNDROME' STRIKES

The following case studies deal more generally with peri-menopause, what is for many a rocky road towards menopause.

## *Iris's story*

**'I DON'T *DO* MENOPAUSE'**

**The Hormone Doctor:** Iris was 50 years old, single and the CEO of a well-known designer label. Her job was demanding, with lots of responsibility, and deadlines and budgets to be met. But since she had started to suffer the effects of peri-menopause, she began to feel despondent. She was overwhelmingly tired and wasn't as motivated in her job as she had been previously. She was worried about getting old, looking old and – worst of all – feeling old. 'Not a good look,' as she put it. Iris asked for my help, proclaiming, 'I don't *do* menopause.'

Iris knew she was approaching menopause but did not know what she could do about it. She had read books on the topic but said she wished she hadn't. She said it was like 'going from blissful ignorance to the grim reaper'. The books Iris had read conveyed the horrors of menopause and advocated conventional HRT as the only option. Fear of ageing, fear of a loss of attractiveness and sexuality, fear of cancer, fear of heart disease, fear of wrinkles, fear of osteoporosis, fear of depression, fear of Alzheimer's – these were the worries driving women to conventional HRT.

Iris's main symptom was excessive tiredness. She had lost her drive and interest in her career. She started questioning her life, what she was doing and if she had made the right career choices and personal decisions. She felt useless. She needed a change but didn't know what to do.

Iris wasn't sleeping well. She would wake in the early morning hours and not be able to fall asleep again until shortly before she had to get up. She only occasionally experienced hot flushes, which she found more annoying than anything else. They didn't really bother her but she didn't like the way she felt and was worried that she was slipping into a mid-life crisis or maybe even depression.

Iris's concerns were justified; things were changing. Iris was peri-menopausal and her 'chi' or 'drive' was waning, along with her hormones. Often, the symptoms of peri-menopause are considerably worse than menopause itself. This is the time of greater change, and the effect on the body and mind can be huge.

Tests of Iris's hormone levels clearly showed that her oestrogen and progesterone levels were fluctuating. She was no longer producing as much of either hormone nor as regularly as she used to. Iris was still menstruating, but that was changing too. I replaced, or rather replenished, the oestrogen and progesterone Iris was lacking in the form of a cream, to be applied daily except when she had her period. All Iris required was a top-up of these hormones, since her ovaries were still functioning, albeit insufficiently. As time goes by and Iris's ovaries cease to function, her hormonal requirements will change, but these can be addressed every step of the way until she reaches menopause.

**The Nutritionist:** Because Iris's energy levels were low, her eating habits were very erratic. She was relying on coffee, tea and far too much chocolate to keep her going throughout the day, and these very habits were exacerbating her already precarious emotional situation.

I took Iris in hand and pointed out that she really needed to take stock of her eating habits, as she was undermining the full potential of the bio-identical hormone replacement treatment by not nourishing herself appropriately. It is not uncommon for women in this situation to neglect themselves, and particularly their eating habits.

Iris's symptoms centred around poor energy levels and mood swings. I recommended that she follow a blood-sugar-balancing program by eating regularly, eating little and often, and cutting down substantially on 'uppers' such as caffeine and sugar, which ultimately deplete you of the very nutrients you need to stay on top of things.

I recommend the same to any woman whose energy levels have dropped considerably: incorporate energising foods into your weekly diet to provide complex carbohydrates, as well as iron, zinc and B vitamins.

Complex carbohydrates are grains that have not been broken down into refined versions of their former selves (for example, brown rice and wholemeal bread, rather than white rice and white bread).

B vitamins are involved in the production of energy at a cellular level, and should be consumed on a daily basis to ensure continuous energy. All complex carbohydrate foods, including pulses, lentils and beans, are rich sources of the B-complex range of vitamins.

Iron is essential for carrying oxygen and other nutrients in the blood to wherever they are needed, and zinc is vital for more than 200 enzyme processes throughout the body, including the production of energy from protein foods (from both animal and vegetable sources).

## Energising megafoods

- brown rice, pearl barley, rye, buckwheat (delicious in pancakes) and udon noodles – these grain-based foods provide all the B vitamins for energy
- sweet potatoes, parsnips, turnips and raw carrots
- spinach, asparagus, blackberries, apricots, apples, parsley, watercress and beetroot – all great sources of non-constipating iron – a far better option than iron supplements
- lentils (rich in iron and B vitamins), chickpeas, butter beans, garbanzo beans, kidney beans (also rich in phyto-oestrogens) and black-eyed peas – pulses are one of best sources of slow-release energy: include them daily in salads, soups and casseroles

## Helpful herbs and spices

The following herbs and spices provide the right kind of energy-producing stimulation and don't have any of the addiction problems that come with caffeine and sugar.

- ginger
- paprika
- turmeric – also fantastic for your immune system
- cumin
- cayenne pepper
- coriander seeds – also fantastic for cleansing the colon
- licorice – but *not* the sweet variety sold in candy stores; go for deglycerinised licorice, found in health food stores, either as a supplement, a tea, or in a chewable version

## Supportive supplements

Iris also needed supportive supplements, as her eating habits had been erratic for some time and she was obviously nutrient-deficient. The following table provides options for boosting your own energy levels.

Remember that you should always start with the foundation of a good-quality multinutrient and then add specific energy-boosting supplements, such as CoQ10, iodine (to support the thyroid and thus metabolism) and other known stimulating herbs, such as guarana, yerba maté and green tea extract.

| Supplement | Daily dosage | Good for . . . |
|---|---|---|
| CoQ10 (must be taken in oil form, as this is the only way it can be absorbed) | 60 milligrams (anything less than this is a waste of time) | Energy production at a cellular level; excellent antioxidant |
| B-complex (B1, B2, B3, B5, B6, B12, folic acid and biotin) | 25–50 milligrams of each of the six B vitamins, 400 mg folic acid and 150 mg biotin | Essential for energy production, balancing mood, concentration and focus |
| Calcium | 150 milligrams | Energy production and bones |
| Magnesium | 300 milligrams | Energy production, muscle relaxation and stress management; supports thyroid function |
| Manganese | 25 micrograms | Important for the breakdown of carbohydrates into glucose for energy, as well as for bone health; also an antioxidant |
| Zinc | 50 milligrams | Boosts immunity; important for metabolism of protein foods |
| Selenium | 200 micrograms | Potent antioxidant and thyroid-supporting nutrient |
| EFAs (essential fatty acids) – must include omega-3 in the form of EPA and DHA in a 2:1 ratio (e.g. 300 milligrams EPA to 150 milligrams DHA) | 600 milligrams | Omega-3 is broken down into bio-available sources to be more readily absorbed – known as EPA and DHA; the correct ratio ensures that each cell is provided with the essential fatty acids vital for allowing nutrients into the cell and toxins and natural waste products out of the cell. Low-fat diets often unwisely restrict the intake of these essential fats |
| Omega-6 | 300 milligrams | Must be taken in the correct ratio with omega-3s to provide your body with the right balance; taking omega-3s on their own in the long term will throw off the balance that the body needs |

**The Hormone Doctor:** After two months of treatment, Iris felt better but still not on top of the world. The hormones were certainly making an improvement but she was still questioning her life and future. She was definitely performing better at work, but on a personal level there were still things worrying her.

She was seriously considering a change of work environment and maybe even moving to another country. However, her decision did not have to be imminent and on the whole she felt there was an improvement in her attitude and energy levels, and she was more positive than before. She was happy to wait before she made life-changing decisions because she did realise that her fluctuating hormones were contributing to her erratic moods and energy levels. She was now ready to wait until she felt more stable and confident about going through menopause and no longer had to fear the grim reaper.

**The Nutritionist:** While Iris's energy levels had greatly improved with the bio-identical hormone treatment and the nutritional changes, her moods were still waning. Just because there is an improvement in energy levels does not always mean there is an improvement in mood.

So we worked together on improving her mood by including those foods that have an uplifting effect. Try several of the following uplifting megafoods for yourself and see.

## Uplifting megafoods
- cottage cheese, turkey, fish and bananas – contain tryptophan, a known mood-enhancer
- brown rice and oats – boost serotonin, the happy neurotransmitter; eat with a small amount of protein to prevent the drowsiness they can cause if eaten on their own

- seaweeds and wild rice (which is actually a seaweed, not a grain) – rich in iodine, which is essential for our metabolism, energy production and weight management; sushi wrapped in nori seaweed is a good place to start
- flaxseed oil – use in salad dressings, as this improves your mood all round
- chocolate – it can be good for us, but only the cocoa contains antioxidants and is mood-enhancing, so eat good-quality dark chocolate only; treat it like fine wine – a little goes a long way and should be savoured
- oily fish and seafood (sardines, mackerel, salmon and trout) – the omega-3s in these fish are vital for the absorption of other brain- and mood-boosting nutrients; without sufficient omega-3 in the diet, the mood will inevitably drop (vegetarians should consume nuts, seeds and their oils on a daily basis to ensure they are getting adequate amounts of omega-3 and -6 essential fatty acids)

## Supportive supplements

If you need more than just a little lift, try adding some of the following mood-boosting nutrients. I recommend that you consider working with a nutritionist on these types of supplements, however, as a nutritionist's experience will help you to select those that are best for your type of problem, whether it be depression, low mood and/or anxiety.

| Supplement | Daily dosage | Good for . . . |
|---|---|---|
| Choline | 25 milligrams | Cognitive function and memory |
| GABA (gamma-amino-butyric acid) | 100 milligrams | Natural mood-enhancing neurotransmitter that increases dopamine levels |
| St John's wort (but avoid using it if you suffer from anxiety, as it can exacerbate it) | 300 milligrams hypericin extract (capsules or tablets) each morning with breakfast; keep to a single dose if combining with 5-HTP | Mood elevation; it takes several weeks for the effects of St John's wort on serotonin to accumulate, so taking it regularly is vital |
| 5-HTP (5-hydroxytryptophan) | 100 milligrams in the morning and optional in the evening – may induce sleepiness, in which case take 200 milligrams at night | Precursor of serotonin – often low in those who suffer from depression; helps maintain emotional stability and reduce sleep disturbance |
| SAME (S-adenosylmethionine) | 200 milligrams twice daily on an empty stomach; may be increased to 400 milligrams three times daily – once a balanced mood is attained, cut back gradually to a maintenance dose; should be taken with 50 milligrams each of B6 and B12, and 200 milligrams of folic acid | Helps produce serotonin and dopamine, accelerating mental clarity, and natural sense of wellbeing; the longer it is used, the more beneficial the results |
| EPA/DHA | 300 milligrams EPA : 150 milligrams DHA (this ratio is optimal for regulating mood and enhancing cognitive function, and is superior to an EPA-only supplement) | Important for mood enhancement, cognitive function and general wellbeing, as well as the absorption of all other nutrients related to brain neurochemistry |
| Zinc | 50 milligrams | Works with vitamin B6 in mood elevation, prevention of depression, increased cognitive function and memory |

**The Hormone Doctor:** I could go on forever with examples of how supplementation with bio-identical hormones changes women's lives. Because of the bad press the synthetic hormones have had, many women have decided to go the 'natural' way and would not consider taking any form of HRT. I have women coming to me saying, 'I don't want to take HRT, but I will take the natural HRT.'

This is one of the first misconceptions I have to sort out. Women come to me because they didn't want to take HRT and they want an alternative. I often note their disappointed faces when I say to them that natural HRT *is* hormone replacement. I then go on to explain the difference between synthetic hormones and 'natural' or bio-identical hormones, why bio-identical hormones may be essential for us and why we should steer away from the synthetic or artificial hormones. I don't ever want to persuade anyone – it must be a patient's individual decision – but I do want to advise my patients so they can make that decision an informed one. Most patients who have come to me have happily accepted treatment with bio-identical hormones. It has made sense to replace what is missing with exactly the same substance – in this case, with our own individually tailored bio-identical hormones and not synthetic ones.

## Angela's story

### 'EVERYTHING'S FALLING APART AND I'M NOT COPING'

**The Hormone Doctor:** Like many of my patients, the first thing Angela said upon entering my practice was, 'I don't want to take HRT.'

Angela was 52, petite and neat, and appeared hesitant to talk about herself. Her periods had ceased about two years earlier and she thought she had got off lightly when it came to menopause – she'd had just a few hot flushes. Perhaps her skin had become a little bit drier and she had a few more noticeable wrinkles, but she considered herself lucky compared to some of her friends, who had suffered a lot and had reluctantly gone on conventional (synthetic) HRT.

While I was taking her history, it was apparent that Angela was quite anxious. She explained that she didn't feel like herself: 'I feel as if someone has pulled out the plug and I'm not coping.' Angela was an administrator in a school. She had two children – one had already left home and the younger one was still studying. She was living in the same small town she grew up in, her husband was her childhood sweetheart and she felt very insecure when things changed around her. She went through a bout of 'empty nest' syndrome when her elder child left home and now she was worrying about her second child, who was also preparing to move out.

Angela's relationship with her husband was good, but she had not had intercourse with him for more than six months because she was afraid that it would be too painful. In fact, Angela was working herself into a state. She was worrying about everything: her children, her work, her lack of libido and now also her total lack of self-confidence.

Until recently, Angela had felt that she had her life under control. She was a perfectionist; she didn't like surprises. Everything had to be planned and organised, but now she felt as if her life were in disarray. Her children were nearly independent, she was retreating physically and emotionally from her husband, she had lost her confidence at work and did not know how to help herself. Her own GP had offered her antidepressants and HRT as possible treatments for her anxiety but Angela wanted neither. She was used to helping herself and didn't want to take medication unless she felt it was necessary.

I had a long first session with Angela and realised that she needed a lot of support and counselling. I also explained to her how bio-identical hormone therapy could play a supportive role in what was happening. She was willing to try and, after the necessary tests, I gave her a combination of oestrogen, progesterone and testosterone together in a cream, which could be absorbed through the skin.

It was remarkable how quickly Angela's emotional state improved after she began using the cream. She no longer had that 'empty' feeling and her confidence began to return. After initiating this treatment we had a few counselling sessions, which helped Angela talk about herself and her fears. She then started seeing a therapist and had cognitive behavioural therapy to cope with her bouts of anxiety and incessant worrying. She felt she needed the hormones because they made her feel 'complete' and 'more confident'. She could now slowly let go of her children and resume a sexual relationship with her husband. She was happy about taking something 'natural' rather than conventional HRT.

**The Nutritionist:** Anxiety like Angela's is common in women whose hormone balance is seriously out of whack, but is also treatable through diet and nutrition. I assured her that, providing she concentrate on a dietary regime that included calming foods rather than those that tended to overstimulate, she would feel better within a couple of weeks.

Like so many women who come to my practice feeling they are 'losing control', Angela was consuming more of the sorts of foods that would exacerbate rather than ease her problem – stimulating drinks such as tea (often mistakenly thought of as a 'calming' drink), coffee (which serves only to heighten anxiety in those who are prone to it, increasing the sense of 'losing control' rather than reversing it) and alcohol (to give her 'a sense of confidence' – which it inevitably did *not*). I suggested first that she cut back on these beverages completely, as well as integrate plenty of calming megafoods into her daily diet.

I would recommend the following calming megafoods to anyone who suffers from anxiety, panic attacks or just a general sense of unease and worry.

## Calming megafoods

- dark green leafy vegetables, including curly kale, Savoy cabbage, watercress, as well as parsley, rocket and zucchini (courgettes) – each contains lots of magnesium (which helps in stress management); I also always recommend magnesium supplements, even when the diet is near-perfect
- brown, red Camargue (French) and brown basmati rice – for calming and balancing, and B-vitamins
- porridge oats, semolina and quinoa – make sure you include a variety of these calming grains
- almonds – there is no nut richer in magnesium; soak them for a couple of hours in water or rice milk to make them more digestible, or put them in the blender for a nut 'milk' – delicious!
- eggs – a great source of magnesium as well as choline, which works directly on the neurotransmitters in the brain, helping to balance both your 'get up and go' and your sense of 'calm'
- chamomile, valerian, hops and passionflower (passiflora) herbal teas – they really do calm you down

## Sarah's story

### LUMPY BREASTS

**The Nutritionist:** Sarah was a beautiful red-headed 44-year-old Welshwoman, with three children and predominantly great health. For years, however, she had suffered from 'lumpy boobs', which she found increasingly worrying as she got older. In an initial sense of denial about the prospect of possible breast cancer, Sarah thought that her lifelong diet of red meat and potatoes, along with a more than healthy dose of alcohol, might have contributed to her state and she wanted my help to address this.

Of course, any patient concerned about the risk of breast cancer and presenting with lumpy breasts should see a doctor, so I referred Sarah directly to Marion.

**The Hormone Doctor:** I examined Sarah and she did have very lumpy and dense breast tissue. The examination was uncomfortable for her. It was a week before her period was due – a time when she could barely cope with anyone touching her breasts, they were so sore. At this time of the month, Sarah would often wear a bra to bed for the extra support, and lying on her side was too painful for her. Sarah also found that her breasts changed size and density depending on the time of the month.

I sent Sarah for a mammogram and ultrasound – it is important to have both examinations, as cysts are more easily recognised in an ultrasound, whereas lumps and calcifications show more clearly in a mammogram. As I suspected, Sarah had fibrocystic breasts, which presents itself as areas of dense breast tissue that are hormonally sensitive. The breast tissue would change depending on hormone fluctuations at different times of the month.

This problem can be precipitated by either too much oestrogen or too little progesterone at the right times of the month. I therefore gave her a bio-identical progesterone cream to use from the day of ovulation to the beginning of her period. This helped reduce the breast tenderness and softened the texture of the breasts themselves. I then sent her back to Vicki for nutritional recommendations.

**The Nutritionist:** I explained to Sarah the importance of cutting down her consumption of saturated fat in red meat and dairy products. I suggested that initially she should cut out both red meat and dairy produce, and eventually replace these altogether with organic white meat and fish, along with goat's, rice and almond milks.

Sarah would also benefit from cutting out all fried foods. When fats are fried, their molecular structure is altered, rendering them more harmful to arteries, as well as contributing to the overall risk of breast cancer. Rancid fats create free radicals that are damaging to breast tissue and to other organs throughout the body.

This is an important point for all women of peri-menopausal and menopausal age. Saturated fats, found in red meat and dairy produce, tend to elevate cholesterol levels. Since some cholesterol that is produced in the liver may be converted into oestrogen, this increased cholesterol may affect the levels of oestrogen circulating in the body. This is one of the reasons why, particularly in women over 40, elevated cholesterol levels are watched very carefully.

Lean proteins should be the major sources of protein for women from the age of 40. Such proteins are found in game birds, fish, seeds, nuts in small quantities (almonds, walnuts and hazelnuts are best as they have the lowest saturated fat content of all) and beans and pulses, which contain no saturated fat.

I suggested that Sarah introduce vegetables rich in phyto-hormones (celery, chicory, fennel and dill – see page 100 for more) into her diet before switching gradually over the next eight to 10 weeks from cow's milk to soy, which also contains phyto-hormones, in order to avoid adding too many phyto-hormone foods too quickly before the hormones balanced themselves out. I also explained that the aim with phyto-hormones is to mimic the body's own oestrogens, occupying the receptor sites in hormonal tissues, such as the breast, ovaries and uterus. By the end of the fourth month, I said, she should notice a significant difference in the density of her breast tissue, along with a reduction in lumpiness.

As an additional measure, I gave Sarah a nutritional supplement of DIM (diindolylmethane) – a concentrated form of a compound found in cruciferous vegetables such as broccoli, Brussels sprouts and cabbage, which helps to redress the oestrogen–progesterone imbalance in women with problems of unopposed oestrogen (that is, sufficient or excessive oestrogen but low progesterone). DIM is usually only available by recommendation from a nutritionist or doctor.

After six months, Sarah came back to see me. She had clearly taken on board my suggestions and had noticed, in her monthly breast examinations, that the lumpiness of her breast tissue was definitely reduced. She was thrilled and said she had dreaded going through the rest of her life 'engaged in a touchy-feely every morning in the shower out of sheer fear that another lump had come up overnight'. I assured her that many women have lumps in their breast tissue, that their occurrence is often related to oestrogen imbalance or progesterone deficiency, and can be remedied by restoring those hormonal imbalances. Finally, I reminded her that it was of the utmost importance that she continue to carry out monthly breast examinations and go back to Marion if she was ever in doubt about a 'new lump'.

## Breast-care meganutrients

| Supplement | Daily dosage | Good for ... |
|---|---|---|
| Starflower (borage) oil | 1000 milligrams | Reduces lumpy breast tissue associated with unopposed oestrogen; contains six times more GLA (gamma linolenic acid) than evening primrose oil |
| Magnesium | 300 milligrams | Works with starflower oil in balancing hormones |
| Vitamin B6 | 75 milligrams | Works with zinc to regulate hormones |
| Zinc | 30 milligrams | Works with vitamin B6 to regulate hormones |
| DIM (diindolylmethane) | 100 milligrams | Helps regulate oestrogen and reduces lumpy breast tissue associated with unopposed oestrogen |
| Selenium | 200 micrograms | Protective antioxidant |
| Glutathione | 50 milligrams | Supports liver; potent antioxidant |
| Multiple antioxidant multinutrient, including vitamins A, C and E, zinc, selenium, alpha-lipoic acid, alpha- and beta-carotenes, CoQ10 and glutathione | Dosage varies according to variety of multinutrient; this is an alternative to taking the above antioxidants separately | Helps protect against oxidative damage, free radicals and cancers |

### Foods to avoid

- coffee
- strong tea
- alcohol
- soft drinks (containing aspartame, sugar or other sweeteners)
- salty foods

### Aromatherapy herbs

These herbs and their oils are known to be beneficial:

- clary sage (but avoid this if you are pregnant, as it can increase the risk of miscarriage)
- geranium

Women with hormone imbalances should take care when using aromatherapy oils in massage, some of which may not be safe. Select your aromatherapist carefully, ensuring they are knowledgeable about how herbs can affect hormones, and that they always offer you the proposed oil for a smell-test first. If you tend to turn away, your body is telling you that you don't need or want that particular oil. Adverse reactions are not uncommon, and some women experience acute detox responses, such as migraines and excessive fatigue, to particular oils.

## WHEN THE TWITCH BECOMES AN ONGOING ITCH: THRUSH AND OTHER STORIES

I have seen so many patients in the course of my 25 years of clinical practice, but some situations occur more frequently than others. Thank goodness it is the less severe illnesses that are more common than serious disease. Thrush and cystitis are two conditions that seem to be extremely common, and in women much more often than men.

The symptoms of these conditions can range from mildly inconvenient to severe, but they always need to be taken seriously. Untreated, both thrush and cystitis can become debilitating – not only interfering with your lifestyle, but leading to serious illness. These ailments need to be picked up on and dealt with quickly – they really need their butts kicked straightaway.

Why are we women more plagued with these symptoms than men? Of course, our anatomy plays a role, but so does our intake of hormones and antibiotics. Bacteria and fungi are part of our physiology, and their proper functions are maintained by a delicate pH balance. When pH levels in our bodies shift slightly to more acidic, it can lead to an overgrowth of bacteria and fungi. These bacteria and fungi then become pathogens and, instead of maintaining their beneficial effects in our body, they can cause thrush and urinary tract infections.

Many readers will have had the unpleasant experience of getting thrush after taking a course of antibiotics. Antibiotics are fairly indiscriminate in their antibacterial effects, destroying both good and bad bacteria. This causes a shift in the pH balance and allows for an overgrowth of pathogenic bacteria, which then causes the symptoms of thrush: vaginal discharge, and vaginal itching and soreness. In France it is common practice to prescribe *Lactobacillus acidophilus*, the healthy gut bacteria that we all require, with every course of antibiotics.

Too many women, young and old, suffer from persistent, frequent or chronic thrush. They have used every antifungal cream, suppository or oral tablet you can name, have changed to cotton underwear, stopped wearing tight jeans, and even abstained from intercourse to resolve these problems. All of these actions can help to combat thrush, but only restoring our physiological pH balance will successfully resolve the situation.

This is where balanced hormones and optimal nutrition play a role in combating chronic thrush. The following case history illustrates these points.

## Bella's story

### CONTINUOUS BOUTS OF THRUSH AND 'BRAIN FOG'

**The Nutritionist:** Bella came to me complaining of continuous bouts of thrush, itchy ears and 'brain fog'. In her late 40s, she was clearly in the middle stage of peri-menopause. She had only two or three periods a year, which were very light. 'I just wish the whole thing would finish,' she said.

An intelligent woman, and well aware of her own health, Bella had researched the possible causes of thrush, but was stumped. She had never suffered from thrush before her late 40s, and had no vaginal dryness or pain during intercourse, so she couldn't understand why the thrush was occurring. 'I haven't taken any antibiotics for the last eight or nine years, I don't eat sweet foods – what do you think the problem could be?'

Thrush can occur if bacteria migrate from the digestive tract to the vagina after a woman has consumed an abundance of sweet foods and refined carbohydrates, as these foods feed pathogenic bacteria. It can also occur, however, when oestrogen levels in the body drop, a common complaint for women going through peri-menopause. As I've said, the pH balance in the body, and particularly in the vagina, is a major regulator of good and bad bacteria. In Bella's case, her long-term use of the contraceptive pill may well have affected her delicate vaginal pH.

I referred Bella to Marion so she could address her hormone imbalances before I recommended any dietary changes.

**The Hormone Doctor:** It was obvious that thrush was making Bella's life harder. It was not only affecting her physically, but it was also having repercussions in her relationship, as the condition was exacerbated every time she had intercourse. Bella's sexual desire had waned, which was not surprising since intercourse had become increasingly uncomfortable. This was unpleasant and she was quite embarrassed by it. She had taken countless courses of antifungal medications to ameliorate the problem, but these medications seemed to work only symptomatically and for short periods of time.

I discussed many factors with Bella – her lifestyle, her relationship and issues that caused her stress. She seemed quite depressed about the situation, as she could not work out why this so-called simple problem could not be resolved. I suspected that Bella's recurrent bouts of thrush were due to her long-term use of oral contraceptives. She had never stopped taking the pill because she was terrified of becoming pregnant, having made a very conscious decision early in her life that she did not want children. Her partner felt the same way but, like many men before him, was not ready to have the 'snip', and so all responsibility for contraception fell to her.

I asked if it would be feasible to take her off her contraception for a few months to see if this was the cause of her thrush. I also asked if she would abstain from intercourse for a period of four weeks to allow her vaginal membranes time to heal. Bella reluctantly agreed. She had some insecurity about the latter prospect, as her reduced sexual activity was already causing some friction in her relationship. Her inadequate nutrition also played a role, but Vicki would address this.

Bella did not have a recurrence of thrush in the following weeks, which made her feel confident that she was on the right track. Six weeks later she started being sexually active and to her surprise the thrush did not reappear. Contraception was still a huge issue for her, and so she decided to have an IUD inserted instead of going back on the pill.

**The Nutritionist:** I provided Bella with a list of foods that would help regain the pH balance in her body. Increasing her intake of fresh, raw green vegetables was a must, to help provide vital minerals such as iron, magnesium and potassium, which help maintain an alkaline pH. Most fresh and raw foods are far more alkaline in their raw state, but Bella usually ate only cooked meals (often overcooked, thanks to her work canteen).

I also suggested one of the best remedies I know for dealing with recurrent thrush – including one clove of garlic in a meal every day. The powerful antifungal properties of garlic cannot be underestimated.

I asked Bella to cut out all red meat and dairy foods from her diet, as these are all acid-forming in the body, for the ensuing 12 weeks. I persuaded her to stick to non-caffeinated drinks for the same reason, and gave her a supergreen supplement, which includes powdered wheatgrass, barley grass and most green leafy vegetables, to kick-start the process.

## Recipe for a healthy pH

| Eat more of these (alkaline foods) | Eat less of these (acid-forming foods) |
| --- | --- |
| Green leafy vegetables: watercress; spinach; rocket; kale; cabbage; French, green and runner beans | All meats and poultry, particularly bacon, prosciutto, bresaola and other smoked meats |
| All root vegetables | Sugar in all forms |
| All sprouted beans, peas, nuts and seeds | All fried and processed foods and hydrogenated fats (margarines) |
| Almonds and walnuts | Brazil nuts and hazelnuts |
| Corn, buckwheat, millet, oats, barley and brown rice | White rice and wheat, muffins, bagels and cakes (refined white flour) |
| Bananas, apricots, peaches and nectarines; all berries except strawberries | Tomatoes, capsicum (bell peppers), eggplant (aubergine), strawberries |
| Fresh fish | Shellfish and smoked fish |
| Lentils, split peas and beans (except kidney) | Kidney beans |
| Dulse, wakame and other seaweeds, and miso soup (fermented soy beans) | Tofu, tempeh and soy beans (edemame beans) |
| Herbal teas and vegetable juices | Caffeinated and cola drinks, commercially produced fruit juices |

## CYSTITIS: WHEN THE URGE TO PEE TAKES OVER ALL ELSE

Did you know that there is a difference between a urinary tract infection (UTI) and cystitis?

Cystitis is the inflammation, infection or irritation of the bladder only. Its symptoms are pain, discomfort and a frequent need to urinate. It can take the form of either bacterial cystitis or interstitial cystitis (IC). Bacterial cystitis is usually caused by contamination from bowel bacteria, and most cases of bacterial cystitis are treated with antibiotics. IC has the same unpleasant symptoms but rarely involves the presence of bacteria. Unfortunately, we do not understand the cause of IC, although some suggest it might be an autoimmune disorder, where the immune system attacks the bladder. IC is like an injury to the bladder caused by constant irritation. It is often misdiagnosed and some patients are treated for years with antibiotics before they are told that their urine cultures are free from bacteria.

A UTI might not be restricted to the bladder only. It is a bacterial infection of the urethra, bladder or, in more severe cases, kidneys. One of the most common causes of UTI is known as 'honeymoon cystitis'. I am sure many of us have experienced this. A new relationship, a new passion and then we have to pay for it.

UTIs often affect sexually active women, but the incidence in the elderly can be much higher than in younger people. Once again, hormones play an essential part in maintaining the integrity and elasticity of our pelvic and genital organs.

So many patients in their early 40s who come to me to discuss hormonal issues mention, in the course of our initial consultation, that they have had to take many courses of antibiotics because of recurrent UTIs. There must be hardly a woman out there who has not experienced the similar symptoms of UTIs and cystitis – the frequent need to urinate, the burning and pulling sensation, and the fever, headache and general feeling of being unwell. Evelyn's story is a common one.

## Evelyn's story

### THE VICIOUS CYCLE OF CYSTITIS

**The Hormone Doctor:** Evelyn, a successful businesswoman, was in her early 40s. She led a busy life, as her work involved a lot of travel, but had found a new partner and an engagement was imminent.

Evelyn came to me for a check-up. She wanted an overview of her hormone levels and some advice on how to best look after herself, and how to stay young and attractive for as long as possible. She also wanted to resolve some questions she had never brought up with her GP.

Evelyn had a good constitution, her periods were regular and unproblematic, she never suffered from PMS, she had plenty of energy for her daily routine and contraception was not an issue, as her partner had had a vasectomy after his previous marriage. The bane of her life was her recurrent UTIs, for which she was treated with antibiotics three or four times per year.

Evelyn liked to avoid taking antibiotics, but when the symptoms became intolerable she would succumb to another dose, which disappointingly never gave her complete relief. She told me that her urine had recently been tested to identify any bacteria but came back negative. Evelyn had cystitis but it was not bacterial, it was interstitial (IC). Evelyn experienced bouts of IC, then thrush as a result of the antibiotics. The irritation of the thrush caused severe itchiness and soreness, which at times resulted in a bacterial cystitis. It was becoming a vicious circle.

Evelyn needed to restore the fine pH balance of her genital and urinary tract by using alkalinisation agents such as potassium citrate and changing her diet to include more alkaline foods. It was also important for her to support and strengthen her immune system in expectation of resolving or reducing her attacks of IC.

This was a difficult case, and there is no quick fix for any ch.~~~
or recurrent condition. We can't treat the symptoms alone, we need
to find and understand the underlying cause. The medical fraternity
does not fully understand the cause of IC and there are no suggested
treatments. Supporting the immune system is a good way to start, and
Vicki did a brilliant job helping Evelyn change her nutrition.

**The Nutritionist:** Treatment of interstitial cystitis requires the pH of
urine and other bodily fluids to be balanced, and this can be achieved in
part through diet.

First, I recommended that Evelyn add no salt to her foods, as the
sodium–potassium balance is vital in treating IC. Further, I pointed out
that many foods that are considered acidic are alkaline in their ash (what
is left after foods have been digested). Apples are a perfect example of
this, and are very useful in the treatment of both types of cystitis.

Cranberry juice, on the other hand, is deceptive – if it's made from
simmering fresh cranberries, the resulting juice is highly alkaline and
contains proanthocyanidins (powerful antioxidants) that help to heal
the inflammation of cystitis, as well as prevent growth of the bacteria
responsible for the infection in the first place – the indomitable
E. coli. Commercially produced cranberry juice, however, is a completely
different matter, as the sugars added to the juice to make it more
palatable may be feeding the pathogenic bacteria.

I recommended that Evelyn buy bags of frozen cranberries, add to
them 1 dessertspoon of Manuka honey per kilo, and then blend with
water. Manuka honey is known to ward off E. coli infections; it's found
only in the beehives of southern New Zealand and is widely available
in supermarkets. It is much more expensive than other honeys, but is
worth its weight in gold.

I also recommended that Evelyn drink warm water throughout the day.

This tends to dilute and alkalinise the urine, as warm water requires no 'digestion' as such, whereas cold water has to be warmed in the stomach before being absorbed through the stomach lining, which makes it more acidic when it hits the kidneys. It is well recognised that coffee, tea and alcohol are all acid-producing, so I encouraged Evelyn to steer clear of all three whenever she felt the first signs of her cystitis coming on.

As Marion had asked me to concentrate on boosting Evelyn's immune system, I recommended that she eat a range of fresh shellfish, which is rich in zinc and selenium, the two most important immune-boosting minerals. I gave her several recipes for scallops, oysters and clams – these are considered 'gourmet' foods but are often in abundant supply and are easy to prepare. I also gave her a list of the richest sources of the antioxidant vitamins A, C and E, recommending a selection of fruits for smoothies that she could prepare for breakfast – including peaches, papayas, mangoes, kiwifruit and all the berries. These fruits alone provided her with her daily requirements for vitamin C, as well as ample beta-carotene. I encouraged her to eat avocados almost daily, as they are the most vitamin-E-rich alkaline food.

(For a full list of acid/alkaline foods, see Bella's story on page 90.)

## THE UNWANTED TRIO: CYSTITIS, INCONTINENCE AND VAGINAL DRYNESS

I watch with part amusement, part horror the television ads for 'incontinence pads' that promise us security and confidence while we sway across the dance floor with a handsome partner, all the while peeing in our pants. What is romantic or sexy about that? Don't we deserve better? If it is so common a problem, can we not prevent it from happening to us? Of course we can, but as Western medicine is not prevention-focused but disease-focused, none of us will go to the doctor and ask how we can prevent this (or anything else for that matter) happening.

There are other causes of recurrent cystitis and these are more common in older women. Vaginal dryness reduces the elasticity of the vaginal wall, which can result in UTIs and incontinence. Recurrent or chronic cystitis can be an outcome. Vaginal dryness can also cause incontinence, a common problem for older women, although many women experience vaginal dryness long before they enter menopause. Many are too ashamed to mention this to their doctor or partner. I can't emphasise enough how important it is to have a healthy, moist and elastic vagina. Vaginal dryness can cause minor injuries (for example, tearing the sensitive vaginal membranes during intercourse), which may then lead to bacterial infections.

We can prevent incontinence by preventing vaginal dryness in the first place, and the best way to do this is to ensure that enough hormones are being produced – in particular oestriol and oestradiol, which are vital for a healthy, moist and elastic vagina.

A healthy, moist vagina is essential for a good sex life and for preventing the vagina from atrophy (shrinking). It is essential for preventing urge or stress incontinence because it helps maintain the elasticity of the vaginal wall, which is surrounded by the bladder at the front and bowel at the back. Anyone who has had a mild prolapse (which usually occurs after childbirth) can verify that hormone preparations in the form of creams (oestriol) or pessaries (oestradiol), which help to maintain the integrity of the vaginal walls and mucus membranes, have considerably improved their symptoms.

Vaginal dryness is not uncommon even in younger women. It must be treated to prevent urinary tract infections and all the problems that come with it, as Suzy's story overleaf shows. It needs to be taken seriously – using KY jelly or lubricant is not a solution.

## Suzy's story

**VAGINAL DRYNESS MAKING SEX PAINFUL**

**The Hormone Doctor:** Suzy was 50 years old. She was still menstruating but irregularly and this didn't bother her at all. She slept well, didn't suffer from mood swings and her energy levels were good. She did have some breast tenderness before her periods, as well as some urinary incontinence, especially when she laughed or played tennis, but again, these were things she could cope with. The biggest side effect of her encroaching menopause was a total loss of libido.

Suzy's children were nearly grown up, and she had more time and less stress in her life than ever before. She wanted to enjoy having a more active sex life with her husband but had lost all desire. Intercourse was causing her a lot of discomfort. Her husband was quite patient but this was beginning to cause a problem in their relationship. When they did have intercourse, it was usually very painful for Suzy, especially at the start. The lining of the vaginal wall was thinning and very dry. During intercourse the lining tended to tear and cause a little bit of bleeding. This in turn became very painful and she frequently developed thrush and sometimes even urinary tract infections, which she had never had before. Understandably, Suzy's appetite for sex was very low, since it caused her so much discomfort, which sometimes lasted for days afterwards.

Fortunately, Suzy's case was very simple to treat. I prescribed her a tiny vaginal tablet called Vagifem, which consists of 0.25 milligrams of oestradiol – a bio-identical hormone. Vagifem is readily available in pharmacies and well accepted by most traditional doctors. Fortunately, this is one of the all too rare cases when the pharmaceutical company acknowledges that the bio-identical hormone oestradiol is preferable to the synthetic Premarin. The beauty of this vaginal tablet is that it predominantly works locally, strengthening the vaginal tissues, increasing the elasticity of the vaginal walls and improving vaginal lubrication.

We have learned, however, that taking oestrogens 'unopposed' (without adding progesterone) can lead to negative side effects. So, in order to balance Suzy's hormone treatment, I prescribed a low-dose (50 milligrams) bio-identical progesterone cream, which Suzy could have made up by a compounding pharmacy. I asked Suzy to apply this to her forearms (for absorption through her skin) a week before her period was due or when she started to experience tender breasts (she didn't require it every day since her symptoms were only temporary). This way, she would receive oestradiol for her vaginal symptoms and progesterone to balance the oestradiol and help with her mild premenstrual symptoms.

The results were almost immediate. Suzy had a slight, normal vaginal discharge again, intercourse was no longer painful, she no longer experienced incontinence, and she no longer had any thrush. At the same time, her premenstrual symptoms subsided and she no longer had tender breasts before her periods. What was beginning to become a major problem was so easy to solve.

**The Nutritionist:** Suzy did very well on Marion's bio-identical hormone replacement regime, but with the addition of the phyto-oestrogen-rich megafoods, she really blossomed. I saw Suzy because she was also concerned that her diet should support her peri-menopausal stage. She already had a clean diet, but she wanted to improve on it, especially now that she had time to focus on herself.

I advised Suzy to include all of the following megafoods containing phyto-hormones. I would suggest that you select several for yourself and add them to your meals regularly.

## Phyto-oestrogen megafoods

- fennel, celery and chicory
- buckwheat, rye, barley and brown rice
- sesame seeds, linseeds, caraway seeds and sunflower seeds
- sprouted seeds – including alfalfa (but not if you suffer from lupus, a chronic autoimmune disease, which is aggravated by these)
- mung beans and chickpeas
- garlic and onions (especially red onions)
- yams
- organic soy-based products, such as tofu, tempeh and miso

## Helpful herbs

These herbs play a particularly important role, as they also contain phyto-oestrogen compounds.

- dill
- sage
- red clover
- parsley
- cinnamon
- nutmeg
- fennel seed
- hops (in beer)
- sarsaparilla – great as a tea, not as a fizzy drink

## Supportive supplements

The following supportive supplements can be beneficial for all aspects of menopause.

| Supplement | Daily dosage | Good for ... |
|---|---|---|
| Vitex agnus-castus | Either 10–15 drops or 2 capsules, twice daily | Naturally balances oestrogen and progesterone |
| Black cohosh (most effective in tincture form rather than tablets) | As above | Reduces hot flushes |
| Sage | As part of a total menopausal combination, or 250–300 milligrams | Reduces hot flushes |
| Red clover | As a tea, several times daily, or a 250–300 milligram capsule, once or twice daily | Balancing moods |
| Panax ginseng (Chinese ginseng) | These vary enormously, depending on the source, and the strength; choose a good-quality tincture, and take between 5–20 drops once to three times daily, or drink tea made from the dried root | Helps manage stress and increase energy levels, balancing all hormones, not just oestrogen and progesterone |

All of these foods, herbs and supplements affect women differently. What works for your best friend isn't necessarily going to work for you. You need to try each in turn to determine what is best for you.

## WHEN HEADACHE RULES

How common headaches are. Who has not suffered from some kind of headache? The history of headaches could easily provide the subject matter for a whole book or even a series of books. But since our focus is on hormones, let's look at those headaches that are hormone-related.

I have had so many patients who are migraine-sufferers. Some first experienced migraines during puberty, others much later, in their mid-30s, and still others were hit with their first migraine onslaught in their peri-menopausal and menopausal years. Then there are those who complained of having headaches most of their life but reported that the pain stopped when they entered menopause.

So what do we do when headaches begin to rule our life?

## *Lubianna's story*

### CHRONIC MIGRAINES 'TAKING OVER MY LIFE'

**The Nutritionist:** Lubianna, an American in her mid-50s, came to me complaining of chronic migraines. She was already post-menopausal and had not had a period for at least four years. She had noted, however, that the migraines would start at roughly the same time each month, as though she were still experiencing a menstrual cycle. These migraines were so severe that she would suffer from disorientation, extreme dizziness and nausea, and would see an 'aura'. Lubianna would usually be forced to retire to bed for one or two days; she was unable to tolerate any light and would have little or nothing to eat. She was aware that her headaches had been growing steadily worse since the birth of her children 12 and 14 years earlier, and that they were beginning to interfere with her responsibilities and involvement as a mother.

Lubianna was also seriously overweight, having always battled food addictions and carbohydrate cravings. She had already been to see me several years earlier, as she had been diagnosed as borderline diabetic by her doctor, and told to 'get to grips' with her eating habits before he was forced to put her on insulin. While Lubianna had drastically improved her eating habits, her years of yoyo dieting had clearly interfered with her metabolism and hormonal balance generally, and her ability to lose weight had diminished dramatically. She had always said, 'If I could just lose some weight, I know I'd feel better,' but now this had changed to, 'I don't even care about the weight any more. I just want to deal with the migraines; they are taking over my life.' I decided to refer Lubianna to Marion, as I realised that Lubianna was suffering from a hormone-based series of problems.

**The Hormone Doctor**: It was clear to me that Lubianna's migraines were a direct result of an oestrogen deficiency. She had never suffered from migraine headaches before menopause and it was no coincidence that the two came together. Although she was not suffering from hot flushes, she was certainly suffering from sleep disturbance, which is a clear indicator of oestrogen deficiency. Sleep deprivation, in turn, was exacerbating her migraines.

Headaches – especially migraines – are often caused by the constriction of blood vessels in the head. I prescribed Lubianna a combination of oestradiol and progesterone, as both hormones have a vaso-dilatory effect (helping to dilate the blood vessels to achieve a better flow). The progesterone also has a relaxing effect, which helps induce sleep.

Lubianna had many problems – weight was her big one, but severe headaches made her feel tired and depressed, and she then lacked the motivation to fix things. She needed to address all her problems, and when she found some relief from the headaches through hormone treatment, she became more energised and motivated to do more for her overall health and wellbeing. She was ready then to take on board Vicki's advice.

**The Nutritionist**: Dealing with headaches through changes in diet can be very successful, once food intolerances have been eliminated.

I addressed Lubianna's tendency to snack on carbohydrates by suggesting recipes for healthy snack bars made from jumbo oats, millet flakes and quinoa, with ginger and cinnamon for natural sweetening. These bars would introduce some more protein into her diet, which would help to balance her blood sugar levels, extreme fluctuations of which can often exacerbate, or even cause, headaches.

One of the main points for Lubianna was the importance of fibre in her diet. Constipation increased the amount of oestrogen metabolites (the results of oestrogen metabolism) and toxins re-absorbed into her system, and this was contributing to her headaches. The fibre from whole grains helps regulate the bowel and prevents high blood pressure. Increased blood pressure is often associated with headaches and migraines, as is the constriction of arteries – particularly those leading up to the cranium and brain through the neck.

I recommended Lubianna steep a couple of slices of raw root ginger in a mug of hot water. Drinking a brew such as this helps dilate the blood vessels. For those with a more savoury palate, cayenne pepper, turmeric and paprika also work as vaso-dilators.

The most important factor was to ensure that Lubianna remained properly hydrated. This did not mean simply drinking more water, but also including plenty of hydrating vegetables in her diet, such as cucumber, lettuce and squashes. All of these vegetables are rich in potassium, which helps to combat the dehydrating effects of salt or sodium. Rather than adding table salt to her foods, I suggested Lubianna change to a potassium salt for seasoning, or even better use mixed fresh herbs to add flavour to her meals.

I always look to the essential-fatty-acid status of my patients who suffer from recurrent headaches, as often they are ingesting plenty of natural fluids but, if on a low-fat diet, may lack the essential fats (from fish, nuts, seeds, oils) that allow the absorption of those fluids. Think of plump, full skin (what I describe as properly hydrated skin) – the fatty-acid outer layers of the skin cells have allowed the vital nutrients in, and the toxins out of, those cells. In the same way, when the arteries that carry nutrients and oxygen to the brain lack hydration and essential fats, they become constricted, causing headaches.

Lubianna embraced the nutritional changes and hormone treatment, and after six months she was at last free from her headaches.

# 4

# all about progesterone

## THE HAPPY HORMONE

Progesterone follows oestrogen as the oldest known hormone. All vertebrates produce progesterone, although only in higher vertebrates is it instrumental in the reproductive cycle. Its name comes from PROGEstational STEROidal ketONE.

In humans, progesterone is vital to conception and in sustaining pregnancy, but progesterone can be your best friend at a time when you're not pregnant, as it provides many more beneficial and protective functions to the body.

Progesterone truly is the happy hormone. It is calming; it decreases anxiety and depression and also relaxes us. It helps reduce mood swings and helps us sleep. On the whole, progesterone brings about a sense of peace and tranquillity. It is a natural tranquilliser.

But it gets even better: progesterone has many more positive attributes. It is a natural diuretic, which means it can relieve excess fluid in the body. With hormonal imbalances, particularly when they have too much oestrogen compared with progesterone, pre-menstrual and peri-menopausal women tend to become bloated and retain fluid. Their ankles swell up and often they can no longer wear their rings. Their breasts swell and become tender and painful, and they may feel a general physical discomfort. Even headaches can be a symptom of fluid retention in the brain, all caused by hormonal imbalance. By supplementing progesterone to attain hormone balance, most of the symptoms disappear.

Another important role of progesterone is in building bone. We commonly hear how oestrogen prevents osteoporosis, but there's more to it. While oestrogen maintains bone strength by delaying the loss of bone tissue, it is progesterone, an anabolic steroid, that helps us to build new bone tissue. This is a perfect example of the complementary effect of progesterone and oestrogen: when used appropriately together, they offer the greatest protection against the development of osteoporosis.

Progesterone is oestrogen's companion hormone, and they work to balance each other. The loss of hormonal balance is one of the main causes of gynaecological problems such as fibroids, heavy or irregular bleeding, painful menstruation, endometriosis and premenstrual syndrome (PMS). As well as physical effects, women who are progesterone-deficient can suffer irritability, agitation, fatigue and depression. Commonly these women will complain of feeling like Dr Jekyll and Mr Hyde, or no longer recognising themselves. Progesterone is the first hormone to become depleted on our way to menopause. We can experience the consequences of progesterone deficiency at any age, but it is most commonly seen from our mid-30s onwards.

## PROVERA IS NOT PROGESTERONE!

The media and the medical community often talk about 'progesterone' when they are actually referring to Provera. For example, your doctor might tell you that you are being prescribed progesterone to treat heavy or irregular periods, but then give Provera. Provera is a progestin, a chemical substitute for progesterone, but it is *not* progesterone. In other words, progesterone is a hormone and Provera is a drug.

These diagrams of the molecular structure of progesterone (as produced in the body or derived from plants in a bio-identical form) and Provera (medroxyprogesterone) clearly show how different they are.

*Progesterone*

*Provera (medroxyprogesterone)*

Provera was designed by its inventors solely to mimic the effects of progesterone in the uterus – to combat a thickening of the lining of the uterus, known as endometrial hyperplasia, which can lead to uterine cancer – and thus for use as a contraceptive. Provera wasn't designed to provide the myriad other beneficial effects that progesterone has on the body.

Provera may act like our naturally produced progesterone in some ways, but unfortunately it causes many side effects that progesterone does not. Take a look at the list below.

## Differences between Provera and progesterone

| Provera (medroxyprogesterone) | Progesterone |
|---|---|
| May cause birth defects if taken during pregnancy; can cause masculinisation in female foetuses | Sustains pregnancy and the developing foetus; used to prevent miscarriage |
| May cause blood clots, which can lead to cerebral and myocardial infarctions (strokes and heart attacks) | Decreases the risk of blood clots, working with oestrogen to protect us against cardiovascular disease; also normalises blood clotting |
| Causes fluid retention | A diuretic |
| Can cause depression, mood swings and headaches | A natural antidepressant that relieves headaches |
| Can exacerbate diabetes mellitus | Helps maintain normal blood-sugar levels |
| Can decrease bone density (as seen in young women who regularly use an injection of Provera as a form of contraception) | Builds bone, increases bone density and helps prevent osteoporosis |
| Can cause breast tenderness, swelling and pain | Relieves breast tenderness and protects against fibrocystic breast disease |

Isn't this a paradox? Provera and progesterone are virtually opposites in some of their effects, and yet one is used as a substitute for the other. It doesn't make much sense when you see how they differ, and for many women the use of Provera comes with shocking side effects.

So which one would you prefer to be prescribed to supplement a progesterone deficiency?

## PROVERA AND THE 2002 SHOCK

Provera is one of the drugs used in conventional hormone replacement therapy (HRT). It is usually prescribed in combination with Premarin, a synthetic form of oestrogen (see page 51). In 2002, doctors, governments and the public became aware of the risks associated with taking Provera when the results of a Women's Heath Initiative (WHI) study were published in the USA. What a shock it was to hear that in trying to prevent uterine cancer, we were not only increasing post-menopausal women's risk of cardiovascular disease, but also of stroke and breast cancer! 'To take or not to take HRT?' became the question everyone was asking. Surely women shouldn't have to choose between risking uterine cancer and risking a heart attack – all in order to prevent hot flushes and get a good night's sleep. Somewhere along the way we seem to have gone down the wrong track. Have the interests of the pharmaceutical companies been put before women's health?

The benefits of HRT had been promoted for 50 years, so users of HRT and the medical fraternity were in a state of disbelief. The fall-out from the WHI study was severe, not only for the pharmaceutical companies (sales of Prempro, the leading combination pill of Premarin and Provera, plummeted 74 per cent), but also for the users of HRT. The WHI had concluded that 'although hormone therapy is effective for the prevention of postmenopausal osteoporosis, therapy should only be considered for women at the lowest dose and for the shortest duration for the individual woman'. Many of the women using HRT for severe menopausal symptoms who could not find an alternative source of relief (as advised by the US Federal Drugs Administration) remained on HRT, despite the question mark over whether they were increasing their risk of stroke, heart disease and breast cancer.

The FDA ordered new labelling and prescription regulations for the Premarin family of products. The new labels now read, 'When used solely for the prevention of postmenopausal osteoporosis, *alternative* treatments should be carefully considered.'

## NATURAL PROGESTERONE TREATMENT

Long before the drug Provera was marketed, London-based physician Dr Katherina Dalton pioneered natural progesterone therapy in her PMS clinic. In 1953, in the absence of today's technology, progesterone had to be sourced from human placentas and could only be administered via an intra-muscular injection. Dr Dalton had good success with her natural progesterone therapy, but there was one problem – progesterone was absorbed only poorly when taken orally and needed to be injected. The research that followed led to the synthesis of Provera, a substitute for progesterone that could be administered orally. But why do we hear so much about Provera and so little about natural progesterone nowadays?

Natural progesterone therapy has simply been overshadowed by the progestin (synthetic progesterone) marketed by pharmaceutical companies to the medical fraternity. As we have seen, Provera was designed solely to mimic progesterone's uterine effects. It had the benefit of being absorbed by the body efficiently as an oral pill, but it does not fulfil all the other important roles progesterone plays in the body. Now, however, progesterone is available in what is called a 'micronised' form – it can be absorbed through the skin and mucous membranes or taken orally. The upshot is that you can now replace progesterone in your body with the real thing. And if bio-identical progesterone is prescribed in a dosage that occurs naturally in the body, its efficacy, safety and tolerability are second to none.

Women are able to remain on bio-identical progesterone therapy for much longer periods than on conventional Provera treatment.

Armed with an understanding of the difference between Provera and progesterone, you are now able to make an informed choice about how to treat any progesterone deficiency you might experience. You may need this knowledge to discuss your treatment options with your doctor.

But how do you know when you're lacking progesterone and when you may need to treat it? Consider the following case study, where a patient suffered a classic peri-menopausal progesterone deficiency.

## Sharon's story

### MOOD SWINGS: 'PERI-MENOPAUSE IS HELL!'

**The Hormone Doctor:** Sharon practically barged her way into my consultation room. She sat down with a bang, leant over my desk and shouted, 'Peri-menopause is hell! Sort me out. I'm at the end of my tether.' Sharon was a 45-year-old advertising executive with a husband and two teenage children who were slowly losing patience with her unpredictable behaviour. She said that she was experiencing tender breasts, but that she was mostly concerned with her mood swings.

Sharon told me that she was having problems at work. She was irritable with her staff, often for no reason, and when she lost her temper she would also lose control of her behaviour. She only really felt well for one week each month – during the time she had her period and for a few days after. The rest of the time she said she was like 'a teenager with constant PMS'.

Although Sharon had a good sense of humour and could laugh at herself, she was actually feeling desperate. She was a very competent woman, perhaps even a bit of a perfectionist, who now felt out of control.

Sharon cried as she told me that for the first time in her life she felt inadequate; she was losing her confidence and felt afraid.

Sharon said that if she had gone to her own doctor, he would have told her to calm down or maybe to take a holiday; he might have even prescribed her some anti-anxiety pills. But Sharon knew that there was an explanation for her behaviour. Maybe it had something to do with hormones, those nebulous things she knew so little about, despite having heard them mentioned so often in chats with her girlfriends.

I explained to Sharon what I suspected was happening hormonally to her body. I told her that it was likely that she was no longer ovulating every month, and therefore was not forming the corpus luteum cyst that produces progesterone. If she was not producing enough progesterone, she would be missing out on its happy, calming and balancing effects.

Don't forget how effective progesterone is in keeping us happy, calm and balanced. Progesterone has this calming effect because it relieves tension in the body by working as a diuretic (decreasing fluid retention) as well as enhancing GABA (gamma-amino-butyric acid), a major neurotransmitter that calms the nervous system and prevents anxiety.

Once I had taken blood tests, I discovered that Sharon's oestrogen level was relatively high while her progesterone level was almost undetectable. The explanation that she was progesterone-deficient reassured Sharon. Knowing why she felt the way she did – and that it was treatable – was a great relief. She looked at me and asked, 'Am I going to get my life back?'

I prescribed her a progesterone cream she could apply twice a day from halfway through her cycle until the beginning of her period, telling her that it would take at least one cycle before she'd start to notice a difference. She was thrilled that it was as easy as that. And she wouldn't even have to swallow anything! Sharon walked out of my room with a smile on her face.

I reviewed Sharon's case six weeks later. She had used the cream as I had prescribed and couldn't believe the difference it had made. She'd felt an almost immediate response – she felt calmer and her moods had evened out. Along with this, her breast tenderness had been relieved, her anxiety had gone, her patience had returned, and she had been able to take charge of her moods and her life again.

This is not an unusual or an isolated case. There are so many variations of what happens when women are progesterone-deficient or oestrogen-dominant.

---

**Common cries of women suffering a progesterone deficiency**

- 'I feel like Dr Jekyll and Mrs Hyde.'
- 'Help, before my husband leaves me and the children move out. Do something!'
- 'I don't recognise myself any more.'
- 'I don't know what's happened to me.'
- 'I no longer feel in control of my life.'

---

**The Nutritionist:** Poor Sharon. She had really been suffering. Marion had been able to sort out her hormonal problems relatively quickly, but Sharon also wanted to tackle the problem in her own way. An excellent cook, she wanted my advice on how she could best support herself through her diet.

While certain foods are known to help lift people's mood, these very foods can act against people who find themselves easily flying off the handle. In Chinese and Ayurvedic medicine, some foods are recognised to be 'heating foods' – foods that exacerbate or irritate the liver 'chi', or energy. They can be overstimulating, causing anger and irritability. These are the foods I advised Sharon to cut down on.

## Heating foods

- chilli, paprika, turmeric, cayenne pepper and curry powder
- garlic and onion (particularly raw)
- all red meat, especially non-organic red meat, which may contain synthetic hormones
- coffee, tea, chocolate and all caffeinated drinks
- alcohol

Many women in Sharon's position ask me about alcohol, saying that they are unable to tolerate it any more, and that they find themselves feeling aggressive after a few drinks. This is because alcohol has to be detoxified by your liver, and in the peri-menopausal and menopausal years, women aren't able to break it down as effectively as they used to.

Just as importantly, I wanted Sharon to know which foods she should eat to help stabilise her moods. As with Angela (see page 80), I thought Sharon would benefit from including calming megafoods in her diet (see page 83 for a list of these foods).

There is, however, a straightforward rule for regulating your moods: eat complex carbohydrates at least twice a day. This helps boost the neurotransmitters in the brain, which in turn calm you down. If you have adopted a high-protein, low-carbohydrate diet in the quest to remain slim, how great are you really feeling? Are you feeling calm and balanced? If not, I'd suggest including whole grains, pulses and root vegetables in your diet for seven to 10 days, then tell me if you don't feel the difference. While protein is vital for building and repairing the body, particularly in the peri-menopausal years when bone health is of prime importance, it also causes overactivity in the mind when not balanced with sufficient complex carbohydrates, triggering anxiety.

I suspected that Sharon was possibly also low in essential B vitamins, many of which are required by neurotransmitters. B vitamins also support the stress-management department of the body, the adrenal glands. I asked her to cut back to just one coffee per day, preferably in the morning after her breakfast, since caffeine depletes B vitamins but also because it exacerbates irritability and breast tenderness. I sent her for a blood test to measure her vitamin and mineral status. Sure enough, her results indicated that she was low in vitamins B3, B5 and B6. Vitamins B3 and B6 are both essential for balanced brain function and B5, along with vitamin C, is required for optimal adrenal gland function.

There are cases of anxiety, depression and anger that need not be addressed by hormonal adjustment – the following is a perfect example of how nutrition and lifestyle choices can dramatically affect a woman's general sense of wellbeing.

## *Janine's story*

### PERI-MENOPAUSE: 'IN A CONSTANT STATE OF SEMI-PANIC'

**The Nutritionist:** Janine, a beautiful mother of two teenage children, was 47 years old but you would never know it – she looked 10 years younger, with long blond hair and legs to die for. The first time we met, she presented her problems in the very way she stumbled through the door – in a total dither. She was still fumbling in her handbag 10 minutes after she sat down, although I wasn't quite sure what she was looking for. She seemed flustered, anxious and a little irritable.

'I don't know what's the matter with me,' she said. 'I feel like this most of the time, although I don't really have all that much to be anxious about. My children are both saints (as saintly as teenage children can be), my husband is marvellous, but I feel like a nervous wreck. My doctor put me on Prozac, but that didn't seem to help; in fact, if anything it made it worse, so I took myself off it. I don't really want to be on antidepressants. I'm *not* depressed, but I feel in a state of semi-panic virtually all the time.'

Going through the food diaries Janine brought in, I noted that she had a typical diet of the 21st-century 'healthy woman' – high protein, low starch, plenty of salads and vegetables, interspersed with rather a lot of black ('I don't do dairy') coffee, and sneaking in regular squares of chocolate (dark chocolate only) to keep her going later in the day.

As we saw with Sharon's story (see page 112), while protein foods are vital for rebuilding and repairing the body, particularly in the peri-menopausal years when bone health is of prime importance, they also stimulate the neurotransmitters in the brain, causing overactivity or hyperactivity of the mind when eaten exclusively. I suspected that Janine was possibly low in essential B vitamins, many of which are required to calm the neurotransmitters and create a more balanced sense of wellbeing, as well as support the stress-management department of the body – the adrenal glands.

I asked Janine to cut back to just one coffee per day, preferably in the morning, after her breakfast, and I sent her for a blood test. Her results showed that she was indeed low in vitamins B3, B5 and B6, which are essential for balanced brain function and optimal function of the adrenal glands.

I recommended that Janine add some complex carbohydrate to her daily diet, to provide food sources of B vitamins, including quinoa, brown rice and couscous in her salads, and also gave her a B-complex supplement, with additional adrenal support including B5, zinc and magnesium. As she was reluctant at first to add the starchy carbohydrates, in case she gained weight, I suggested she should try it for two weeks to see if the foods, along with the supplements, made any difference. I also recommended that she drink passionflower (passiflora) herbal tea in the evening, as an alternative to chamomile, which she loathed.

The changes to Janine's diet did have a noticeable effect and she felt significantly calmer. 'I can't believe that just employing these simple measures has made so much difference,' she said during her next consultation. I pointed out that this is one of the common problems I see in women of all ages these days – in the quest to remain slim, they cut out one of the most important food groups, complex carbohydrates, and leave themselves climbing the walls.

## *Tina's story*

### PERI-MENOPAUSAL ACNE: 'I'VE GOT HIDEOUS BREAKOUTS'

**The Nutritionist:** Tina is a favourite client of mine – she has been coming to see me for years, and I have seen her through two pregnancies from the pre-conception stages. Now 38 years old, she came to me recently with a bad case of acne. Tina had always had beautiful skin; in her late teens and 20s she had been a model, so she was particularly distressed by the arrival of these blemishes. 'I don't eat chocolate, I never eat fast or junk foods, and yet I've got spots all over my back, and these hideous breakouts on my face – help!'

After running a blood test, we determined that she was possibly entering a relatively early peri-menopause. I recommended that Tina drink soy milk on her cereal and cut out coffee altogether for the next three weeks. Coffee is a known stimulant, and its effects can be exaggerated when hormones start to get out of balance. More importantly, I wanted to see if she responded well to the soy milk, and to ensure that she didn't have any intolerance to it. (Some women find that soy products can have adverse affects if introduced too quickly.) After one week, I recommended that Tina also buy some fresh miso soup (fermented soy with brown rice or barley), and have this as an afternoon snack in place of anything sweet.

After the three weeks, Tina was feeling better and her skin was improving. In helping to rebalance her declining hormones, the phyto-hormones in soy milk and miso were already helping to clear her skin. I pointed out that balancing her hormones would help to stimulate collagen production, and that eating such foods and redressing the imbalance would have the longer term benefit of helping to plump up her skin – an added bonus!

Several months later, Tina's skin had cleared completely and her confidence was restored. She decided to save coffee for special treats only, as she realised that a lot of her anxiety had been related to the quantities of coffee she had been knocking back. She is now acutely aware of the importance of food and nutrition at this changing stage of her life.

---

### Did you know . . . ?

Clinicians are reporting that they are seeing more and more women who are experiencing the unpleasant hormonal symptoms that come with the onset of peri-menopause in their late 30s rather than in their 40s.

## POST-NATAL DEPRESSION: WHEN THE BABY BLUES TURN BLACK

Most of us know what it's like to get the blues – waking up with a black cloud over our heads, not wanting to face the day or having to push ourselves to get through it. Women may notice that these feelings can be cyclical, and that this sort of depression usually occurs two weeks before their period. Realising that this is part of being premenstrual can help us to grin and bear it because we know it will pass.

Other, longer lasting forms of depression can be devastating, however. Post-natal depression is one form that can severely affect women and their families. There can be nothing worse than having experienced a wonderful pregnancy, one full of joy and expectation, only to be overcome with despair and anxiety after the birth. In some cases the new mother is riddled with guilt because she does not feel 'happy' about her baby's arrival. She may feel inadequate, insecure and overwhelmed, and the father or other family members may have to take over caring for the baby while she recovers from her birth experience.

It is commonly known that new mothers will often suffer from the 'baby blues'; this usually starts three days after the birth but lasts only a few days. We have a good understanding of why this happens. During pregnancy, the blood is flooded with very high levels of oestrogen and progesterone, but after the birth, the levels of these hormones, especially progesterone, come crashing down to almost nothing. In the case of those suffering post-natal depression, these hormones don't return to their normal levels, and this state may last for years or recur with subsequent pregnancies.

Why is post-natal depression treated with antidepressants, when a major cause is obviously hormonal? Most women are prescribed antidepressants, but often these just take the edge off the despair. They become more capable of caring for their newborn but often do not experience the joys of motherhood and parenting. A common complaint is also a loss of libido, and when they stop their anti-depressants there is not much change. Some of the patients I treat with progesterone or a combination of oestradiol and progesterone report an increase in their feeling of wellbeing and no longer consider themselves depressed. Consider Gina's story, below.

## Gina's story

### POST-NATAL DEPRESSION: TRIED 'EVERY ANTIDEPRESSANT'

**The Hormone Doctor:** Gina was 28 when she first came to see me. She was seeking treatment for her severe premenstrual tension. Two weeks before her period she would become so anxious she could not go out socially – she could barely make it to the supermarket, and even then she'd only make it if her mother accompanied her. She had been prescribed an oral contraceptive pill one year earlier by her GP, who thought it might help with her PMS. Unfortunately it only made her feel worse, and she stopped taking it after three months.

Gina told me that she had a three-year-old daughter, and that she had been feeling depressed since her birth. Soon after her daughter was born, Gina felt unable to cope; she even considered running away and leaving the baby with the father's family. She felt miserable, inadequate and desperate. Gina's depression was so severe that she was referred to a mother-and-child respite centre, which offered help in bonding with and caring for newborns. The sojourn in the respite centre helped, but a doctor there prescribed her the first of many antidepressants. Since that time, Gina had been prescribed 'every antidepressant in the book', which only served to take the edge off her symptoms but never gave her total relief.

It would be nice to think that when a patient is on antidepressants they no longer show symptoms such as anxiety or melancholy, but this was not the case for Gina. She continued to tell me that she was managing well with her little daughter, but complained of having little energy and no real joy in her life except for her child. She had no libido and her relationship with her husband was strained. Gina felt that she had let him down as a wife and that she had been an inadequate mother to their child. She saw little of her friends and did not socialise often. She was starting to rely on her mother as her main companion to an ever greater extent.

Although she had come to me regarding her anxiety-related premenstrual symptoms, it was obvious to me that Gina had never recovered from her post-natal depression. Her symptoms had been numbed somewhat by the antidepressant medication she was currently taking, but not enough to stop the anxiety she experienced before each period. The cause of Gina's depression was most likely hormonal, and isn't this what we should treat – the cause, not the symptoms? She had experienced a progesterone crash after the birth of her daughter; now she had a hormonal imbalance and was not producing enough progesterone during the second part of her cycle. As we saw earlier, this important hormone enhances GABA, a major neurotransmitter that produces a calming effect on the nervous system.

I asked Gina to come off her antidepressants slowly under my guidance. I initially prescribed her daily progesterone in a low dose: 25 milligrams from day 1 to day 14 of her cycle, and then 25 milligrams mornings and evenings from day 15 to day 28. I also suggested she have a session with Vicki to see how changes in her nutrition could aid in her recovery.

**The Nutritionist:** Gina was only too keen to try nutritional supplements, especially when I pointed out that she would get back a lot of the sensations that had been numbed by the antidepressants.

I waited until Gina had reduced the amount of antidepressants to half her original prescription before starting her on 5-HTP (5-hydroxytryptophan, a naturally occurring amino acid), which would help elevate her serotonin levels. Over the next month, as she continued to come off her antidepressants, I marginally increased the 5-HTP dose, which helped to rebalance her mood naturally.

I recommended a supplement with a relatively high dose of vitamin B6 (100 milligrams) and zinc (50 milligrams) to be taken once daily for the first week, and then every morning and evening thereafter. Zinc and B6 are both vital for managing many forms of depression, particularly post-natal depression. Several research papers have shown that women have very low levels of zinc and B6 after giving birth, most likely because these nutrients are passed through the placenta to the baby several days before birth in order to boost the baby's immune system. Zinc is essential for maintaining sensitivity in our taste buds, as well as in appetite regulation – and Gina's zinc levels had been very low when Marion first referred her to me.

I also suggested Gina take 1 gram of evening primrose oil daily, in order to help regulate her hormones nutritionally, and a B-complex supplement to ensure that the high dose of B6 would not throw the other B vitamins out of balance. I suggested that she include plenty of zinc- and B6-rich foods in her weekly shopping basket, including shellfish, chicken, turkey and lots of brown rice.

Gina had been living on a very small selection of foods, as she'd had no appetite, but this returned once the effects of the zinc and B6 kicked in. After two months, Gina said she felt like a new woman – the smile was back on her face, as well as on that of her husband.

**The Hormone Doctor:** Gina responded positively to the progesterone. She was hugely relieved and started to feel calm again. This gave her confidence and she started going out by herself. These feelings of relief and confidence led to pride and, eventually, a sense of joy. After three months, I reduced her dose of progesterone and she only needed to take it in the two weeks before her period.

In Gina's case no antidepressant could – or did – achieve these results. Gina had a hormonal imbalance; she was low in progesterone and all she needed was to replace what she lacked. Gina became a sociable and happy woman again. She no longer relied on her mother and started enjoying her company instead of needing it.

I saw Gina regularly over the next couple of years. I did not need to adjust the dose any further, and after two years she was able to stop using the progesterone cream altogether. By that time her ovaries were producing progesterone in sufficient amounts and no longer needed to be supplemented. She was feeling confident as a mother and wife, and when her daughter started school, Gina took on a part-time job. Gina and her husband decided not to have any more children. They were grateful to have the family life they had and said they didn't want to 'rock the boat'.

This is the beauty of bio-identical hormone replacement therapy: you replace what is needed, fine-tune when necessary, and stop when all is well again.

## FERTILITY PROBLEMS

Women with fertility problems, especially those who have had more than two miscarriages, are often progesterone-deficient. Pregnancy cannot be sustained unless sufficient amounts of progesterone are produced in the first trimester. Progesterone can be safely supplemented through the use of a cream, vaginal suppository or injection. It's important here to underscore the point that you must not take Provera or any other type of progestin (synthetic progesterone) during pregnancy, as they can cause birth defects.

## Julie's story

### FERTILITY PROBLEMS: 'WE WANT TO GET PREGNANT AGAIN!'

**The Hormone Doctor:** Julie was 39 years old when she came to see me. She and her husband had an 11-year-old daughter and they wanted to have another child. Julie was healthy and extremely fit, with good energy levels. She was a full-time wife and mother and played a lot of sport in her spare time. She had been trying for the last four years for another pregnancy. Julie had become pregnant easily with her daughter and couldn't understand why she was having problems now. Her periods were occasionally irregular and twice she had thought she might be pregnant because her breasts had been very tender. Both times, however, her periods arrived, although they were two or three weeks later than usual.

Julie and her husband had both been examined, but no cause could be found for her secondary infertility (that is, infertility after having been pregnant before). Julie had been advised to go to a fertility clinic for IVF treatments, but neither she nor her husband wanted to go down that path.

She had done her homework; she had read that low progesterone levels could cause infertility. Although all her tests had returned normal results, she thought it was worth trying a course of progesterone supplementation. I decided to give her progesterone in lozenge form because she was concerned that the cream would not be absorbed properly due to all the sport she played.

I prescribed her dosage in a way that mimicked her own cycle, ensuring a constant baseline of progesterone in her system so she would not experience low levels at any time except during her period.

Julie tolerated the extra progesterone well, and eight months on she was sleeping deeply, and on the whole was relaxed. Her periods had been very regular while on the progesterone treatment, so when she was late she did a home pregnancy test. And, sure enough, shortly after her 40th birthday, she discovered she was pregnant. Julie went immediately to her gynaecologist and obstetrician, who approved of what she had done; he then took over her treatment and Julie remained on progesterone for a further three months. Julie had an uneventful pregnancy and gave birth to another daughter.

Today Julie is healthy and not on any hormone treatments. She plays less sport than she used to – her schedule is a bit busier these days. She recognises that she is now heading towards peri-menopause. If she has any symptoms in the future she knows which way she'll treat them.

**The Nutritionist:** While Marion was helping Julie take steps towards a successful pregnancy, I focused on topping up the vital nutrients that may have been depleted through her high levels of exercise. I speculated that one of the causes of her inability to become pregnant may have been that her exercise regime resulted in irregular periods.

I also suggested to Julie that she increase the amount of essential fatty acids (EFAs) in her diet, as these are necessary for the proper functioning of all hormones, including those that affect fertility, pregnancy and lactation. EFAs are found in nuts, seeds and oily fish (see the fertility megafoods on page 43).

*Did you know ... ?*

It is more common than people realise for ultra-fit women to have very low levels of body fat. It's necessary to have a healthy level of body fat in order to maintain a pregnancy.

## HORMONAL HEADACHES AND MIGRAINES

Many of us will be familiar with the headaches women get frequently in the middle of their cycle at the time of ovulation or right before their periods. For some women these headaches can be so painful and debilitating that they rule their life. Some are driven into their dark bedrooms for three days at a time. Luckily these cases are not the rule – but they're certainly not the exception either.

Both the headaches that occur at ovulation and those that come on right before a period are caused by a hormonal discrepancy. During ovulation there is an oestrogen surge followed by an increase in progesterone. Most likely the progesterone levels increase too slowly to balance the oestrogen and this disparity causes a relative progesterone deficiency. With too much oestrogen, there is dilation of the blood vessels and there may be fluid retention, which can cause pressure in the brain, resulting in a headache.

The same thing happens with headaches caused just before a woman gets her period: insufficient amounts of progesterone are being produced in the second part of the cycle, which means oestrogen is not in balance with progesterone. Again, this can lead to fluid retention and pressure in the brain.

## HELP FOR SUFFERERS OF HORMONAL HEADACHES

So what can we do? For those who suffer from extremely painful and debilitating headaches, bio-identical progesterone therapy can provide some relief by counteracting the blood-vessel dilation that causes the headache. Many women treated this way can experience significant improvement – either they don't need as much pain medication to cope or they have longer intervals between headaches. It must be said, though, that these patients are never completely cured.

A number of foods are known to trigger headaches and migraines and those containing a compound called 'tyramine' are some of the main culprits. Tyramine is found in all smoked meats, smoked fish and smoked dairy products, particularly when they have been prepared in a commercial smoking house. Other baddies include the tannins found in all red wines (especially in heavy red wine varietals) and tea, as well as caffeine. Sadly, chocolate also contains a fair amount of tyramine, which is why so many people get headaches after enjoying a few pieces of their favourite chocolate.

Citrus fruits are great for most of us, but if you are susceptible to headaches, they are a known trigger. Cheeses of all types are also known to cause headaches – and just think of how many of us eat some kind of cheese every day. If you suffer from headaches and simply accept this as part of your life, think again. Why not look at your cheese, citrus and tyramine-rich food intake? Cutting certain foods out of your diet for a certain period of time is a good way to see if they are responsible for generating your headaches.

Additives, flavourings and preservatives are a no-no for anyone suffering from headaches. The worst of these is MSG – often listed simply as 'glutamic acid' on packaging, which is found in most Asian foods and many processed foods. Sadly, it is also added to a lot of dishes in what are no doubt your favourite restaurants, so you should ask your waiter to ensure that no MSG is added to your meal. In the body, MSG is broken down into aspartate, which has a similar effect to the chemical sweetener aspartame. It can cause anxiety, over-alertness and sleeplessness or insomnia. All in all, we are better off without MSG.

Puberty, peri-menopause and menopause are all times when our bodies are in hormonal disarray, and often these times correspond with when women complain that they are suffering from headaches. These are also times when women are frequently ingesting synthetic hormones. Young girls are put on the pill to regulate their periods, and during peri-menopausal and menopausal years women are often prescribed the pill or conventional HRT to regulate symptoms. Headaches are one of the most common symptoms of hormonal imbalance, either because your body is out of whack or because you have been prescribed synthetic hormones.

Here is the story of someone who suffered from headaches for 11 years before she found relief.

## *Veronica's story*

### HEADACHES AND DEPRESSION: 'MY HEAD IS BURSTING'

**The Hormone Doctor:** Veronica was a 41-year-old part-time teacher as well as a carer for her elderly parents. Veronica had quite a few issues she wanted to discuss, but the main cause for her visit was her headaches. They were causing her to miss work at least two or three days out of every month. Her headaches were cyclical, occurring usually in the week before her period.

In her 30s, Veronica had suffered from PMS and she was prescribed the pill to help with this. Shortly after starting on the pill, she developed headaches and depressive moods. Because of her depression, she was put on Prozac and 11 years on she was seeking help to get off this antidepressant.

In those 11 years, no one ever questioned whether the pill was contributing to Veronica's headaches or mood swings, but you need only read the medication information sheet that comes with the pill to see that headaches and depressive moods can be side effects. The pill can act to relieve these same symptoms, but we need to acknowledge that everyone tolerates medication differently. I was surprised to hear that even though her symptoms never improved, no one had reviewed Veronica's medication. In fact, Veronica had been given the impression that she would be worse off if she stopped taking the pill.

I asked Veronica if she'd be happy to stop the pill so that we could observe exactly what its influence was. She readily agreed and the change was remarkable and swift. After two months without the pill, her moods had lifted and she'd halved her dosage of Prozac. The intensity of her headaches had lessened, and she was feeling more positive about life and better able to cope with stressful factors, such as looking after her parents.

After observing this, I realised that Veronica needed to have progesterone supplementation to further ease her PMS and relieve her headaches. Veronica has been on progesterone cream now for more than a year; she is positive and energetic and only sporadically suffers from headaches. Her PMS and mood swings are now controllable on their own, and she has been able to stop her antidepressant medication altogether.

## Joanna's story

### SLEEP DISTURBANCE AND HEADACHES

**The Nutritionist:** Joanna came to see me six or seven years ago, aged 46, complaining of insomnia, nightmares and disturbed sleep patterns, as well as severe headaches that she thought might be more food-related than cyclic. Having always been a sound sleeper until the previous year or so, she couldn't understand why she should suffer from insomnia now. She was happy in a relatively new relationship and her two children were at university, allowing her plenty of private time and few major stresses in her life. While she had recently started to complain of hot sweats at night, they were sporadic, and didn't necessarily have a direct relevance to her insomnia. She found that her nightmares were sometimes so alarming that she had to get up in the early hours of the morning, leaving her partner asleep in bed, as she was often too anxious to risk going back to sleep.

Joanna had always eaten a well-balanced diet, with a good intake of vegetables and fruit, but it was only on closely inspecting her weekly diet that I found she was consuming large quantities of cheese and other dairy products, and sometimes drank more than her fair share of wine at night. She had been trying to lose a little of her 'middle-aged' weight, and had put herself on a relatively high-protein, low-carbohydrate diet – hence the daily consumption of cheese. I spotted the tendency to consume red wine with the cheese as the possible main culprit for both her headaches and her nightmares.

I recommended that she cut out cheese for three months and include soy milk two or three times per week to help her replenish her apparently falling hormone levels with the phyto-hormones (see pages 70 and 100 for more on phyto-hormone-rich foods). I also suggested that she use silken tofu (fermented soy bean curd) in her breakfast smoothies at least twice a week to begin with, in place of yoghurt or cow's milk. And I recommended a supplement containing calcium, magnesium, valerian and passiflora for her to take at night after dinner to help with her insomnia.

I had considered sending Joanna to see Marion, as some of her symptoms were classic signs of hormone imbalance, but I wanted to determine what, if any, involvement foods had with these symptoms first. It turned out I didn't need to refer Joanna. She phoned me the following month to give me an update on her progress: she hadn't had a headache or a bad nightmare from a few days after our appointment, the night sweats had abated, and as icing on the cake she had lost a couple of kilograms. In fact, her sleep patterns had returned almost to normal, with the exception of a couple of broken nights, when she had 'accidentally' had a cheese risotto and a few cheese straws at a cocktail party.

I pointed out to Joanna the several beneficial factors involved with the changes she had implemented: the soy from the tofu and soy milk had helped to redress the balance of the early stages of the peri-menopause, while the eradication of cheese from her diet had lowered her saturated-fat intake, which probably contributed to her weight loss as well as eased her nightmares. Delighted with the improvements, she decided to leave cheese out of her diet altogether and include soy in some form every day from that point on.

## PREMENSTRUAL SYNDROME: WHEN IT'S 'THAT TIME OF THE MONTH AGAIN'

PMS, or PMT, is basically a collection of different physical, psychological and emotional symptoms that are related to the menstrual cycle. For a woman suffering PMS, the symptoms are fairly predictable and usually occur one to two weeks before her period. Some symptoms are severe and others light; some women suffer greatly while others are barely affected. Some women say that they only have one good week in the month – the rest is misery!

I am sure that all women would attest to experiencing some form of PMS, in the form of aching legs, food cravings, bloating, head-aches, tender breasts and moodiness, to name just a handful of symptoms. Many women experience a 'Jekyll and Hyde' situation, with their moods fluctuating severely, or they have such debilitat-ing cramping or headaches that they cannot go about their ordinary daily activities. Women whose PMS severely affects their quality of life need treatment.

When PMS is so severe that it is considered disabling, it has its own psychiatric name: premenstrual dysphoric disorder (PMDD). And although the name contains within it the cause of the disorder, once again the common approach is to treat it with antidepressants. (It would be nice to think that the pharmaceutical companies could be a little more inventive than to promote antidepressants as the panacea for so many conditions!)

## *Sandra's story*

### SEVERE PMS: 'I'M OUT OF CONTROL'

**The Hormone Doctor:** Sandra, a 43-year-old lawyer, had read in a newspaper article about my work, but was still sceptical about what I could do for her. She had given up on a solution for her hormonal problems after trying a range of treatments that didn't work.

Sandra told me that she'd had problems with PMS since her early 20s. She had every physical and emotional symptom in the book, from mood swings to heavy, painful periods. Sandra said that her 'hormones were raging', and now she felt that things were becoming worse again after a short respite during her 30s.

Sandra used very strong words when describing her premenstrual state, saying that she felt 'a deep anger, and could kill'; at other times she felt deep depression, which verged on suicidal. Sandra did not use these descriptions lightly. She told me that she felt 'as if something is dragging me down and I can't get lifted. It feels physical and emotional and I'm just waiting for relief while the pain gets worse'. Her symptoms were always cyclical, with a climax at the time of her period. She was an astute and articulate woman who was now also becoming anxious and worried. She had started experiencing sleep disturbances.

Of course, Sandra's severe mood swings were affecting her life. She had managed to keep things fairly stable at work, until recently when she had behaved inappropriately and 'exploded'. Her colleagues told her that 'she was not being herself', and Sandra was referred to a counsellor. This loss of control was scary for Sandra, as professionally this was a no-go zone. On a private level, however, she cut herself a bit more slack, recognising that her mood swings were not under her control.

Sandra had been on the pill during her 20s and again when she was 38, but it had only made her feel 'crazier'. She used food for comfort when she had bouts of depressive moods and liked to binge on bread and butter; she also constantly snacked on chocolate, but this did not affect her weight, only her moods. Sandra was in a great deal of physical pain, only having a few 'good days' out of every month. She had been on mefenamic acid for the past 10 years to control her period pain, and had been taking Prozac for the last two years.

Someone reading this might suppose Sandra to be a psychiatric case, and there is an argument for this. There was a family history of depression, and Sandra experienced her first depressive mood when she was 13. But life is not simple and people rarely fit into neat boxes for diagnosis. I could not assume that Sandra was only 'hormonal' or only needed psychiatric treatment. Symptoms often overlap to the point where it is difficult to tell what is the cause and what is the effect.

My impression of Sandra was that she was an intelligent, independent woman who was suffering as her 'hormones' were taking control and driving her 'crazy'. All of this was affecting her life, especially professionally, and she was beginning to lose confidence in herself.

I felt I had to respond immediately. She was on the appropriate treatment if the causes were psychiatric: she was already taking an antidepressant; she was on high doses of magnesium, which helps to release tension; and she practised yoga daily. All of this was making a difference, but nothing had been done to balance her hormones, which Sandra still thought were her main problem, since her symptoms were always cyclical and always climaxed at the time of her period.

I decided to prescribe progesterone cream, which Sandra could apply from day 14 of her cycle to day 3 of her next – coinciding with the worst of her emotional symptoms and her heavy and painful period.

Sandra is still a new patient of mine, but after a week on the progesterone treatment she sent me a lovely card, saying that she was feeling particularly well. She had been having 'good days' since using the cream. She did remark that it might be a 'psychological effect', but that she felt much more confident now about finding a treatment that could tame her 'raging hormones'.

**The Nutritionist:** Sandra's case was so severe that Marion asked me to put together a nutritional plan before I had even seen her. Based on Marion's clinical notes, I recommended that Sandra take 50 milligrams of zinc and 25 milligrams of vitamin B6 daily. These nutrients would help address the emotional side of Sandra's PMS symptoms, as this combination has been well documented as an effective treatment for 'menstrual madness'.

In addition, I suggested that Marion prescribe 5-hydroxytryptophan (5-HTP), an amino acid that contributes to the formation of serotonin. Serotonin is a neurotransmitter found in the parts of the brain that affect conscious thought, mood, emotions and memory. Maintaining a constant serotonin output is vital for a sense of wellbeing.

I also suggested a supplement of starflower oil. This oil, extracted from the herb borage, provides the richest source of omega-6 fatty acids, which help with managing breast tenderness and other PMS symptoms such as bloating, constipation and diarrhoea. Starflower oil is six times more potent than evening primrose oil, and has been found to be far more effective in the management of PMS.

Both caffeine and alcohol can aggravate not only fluid retention but also mood swings, anxiety and feelings of self-loathing. It is for this last reason that I recommended that Sandra observe a 'clean' diet during the 10 days before her period – no toxins, no additives, no irritants and no stimulants. A clean diet means eating only fresh fruit and vegetables, fresh fish and light poultry (no red meat), and plenty of raw unsalted nuts and seeds. In fact, I even encourage some of my patients to eat a raw-food diet, as this is the purest approach to consuming highly absorbable, readily available sources of minerals and vitamins that help to eliminate the symptoms of PMS.

After providing this urgent nutritional plan, I did see Sandra in my clinic. Once her mood was elevated with the help of the progesterone cream, she was keen to take on board my advice and viewed the nutritional plan as a way to regain some control over her health – this was something she could *do* for herself.

## What to do about those PMS cravings

In the 10 days before their period, many women find they crave either salty or sweet foods – not, as you might think, for comfort but to replace the minerals that are depleted as our oestrogen and progesterone levels change leading up to menstruation. The most common craving is for chocolate – but why? The reason is that cocoa is rich in magnesium, which helps to relax muscle tissues throughout the body. With the all-too-familiar cramping that occurs (sometimes severely, as in Sandra's case) just before and during menstruation, it is little wonder that chocolate becomes so appealing. It is important to understand, however, that it is the high cocoa content (75 per cent or more) that delivers the magic magnesium, but the more commercial varieties of chocolate are simply laden with milk products and sugars.

Those who don't crave chocolate often find themselves dreaming of salty or pickled foods, as our sodium–potassium balance changes with our oestrogen and progesterone levels. This is what causes the 'fluid retention' associated with PMS – puffiness of the ankles, fingers, thighs or knees. Ironically the more salty or pickled foods you eat, the worse the puffiness becomes and the greater your cravings for more of the same – it's a vicious circle.

## Foods for combating PMS symptoms

Anaemia and related fatigue (including 'heavy legs') is a common complaint during menstruation, since between 15 and 30 milligrams of iron are lost during each period. Iron replacement through food is vital. It is a good idea to start increasing your intake of iron-rich foods four to five days before your period, to ensure you have adequate stores. Animal sources of iron are more readily absorbed in the body than vegetable sources, so a combination of both is required to maintain blood levels. This is why vegetarians in particular suffer from post-menstrual anaemia and why some may require an iron supplement.

Remember, too, that iron requires vitamin C for its absorption. As we do not store vitamin C in the body, we need to ensure that we include sources of it in our diet every day. Consult the lists of iron-rich and vitamin-C-rich foods on the following page.

Omega fatty acids are also vital for the prevention of PMS symptoms. Omega-3 and -6 are both important for the production of oestrogen and progesterone, and a lack of either in the diet will inevitably result in aggravated PMS symptoms. Omega-6 can relieve the breast tenderness and lumpy boobs (fibrocystic breast tissue) that occur in many women before menstruation, while omega-3 helps regulate the fluid retention and uterine contractions that cause period pain. Although oily fish is an excellent source of omega-3, it is important *not* to eat smoked fish before your period, as this will lead to increased fluid retention and weight gain.

## The anti-PMS food rules

Eat fewer salted and pickled foods, such as:

- potato crisps
- packet snacks
- roasted salted nuts
- soy sauce and tamari
- vinegars and pickled vegetables
- bacon, prosciutto and Parma ham
- smoked fish and smoked meats

Eat more potassium-rich foods, such as:

- fresh fruit juices
- bananas, apricots and prunes
- green leafy vegetables
- whole grains such as millet, buckwheat, barley and rye

Eat more iron-rich foods, such as:

- calf and chicken livers, and oxtail
- sesame seeds and tahini
- dark green leafy vegetables such as kale, watercress, rocket, parsley and spinach
- raisins, apricots and prunes

Combine iron-rich foods with vitamin C-rich foods, such as:

- kiwifruit, papaya and mangoes
- citrus fruits
- capsicum (bell peppers), tomatoes and potatoes
- all green vegetables and salad leaves
- fresh fruit and vegetable juice

## PMS-busting herbs

| Herb or tincture | Good for ... |
|---|---|
| Cyanara or artichoke extract | Reduces fluid retention |
| Nettle tea | Natural diuretic and high in potassium |
| Dong quai tea and tincture or as a Chinese herb to be boiled | Relaxes uterine muscle and aids in hormonal regulation |
| Ginger (fresh, powdered and as a tea) | Reduces inflammation that causes painful periods |
| Black cohosh tincture | Relaxes muscle spasms |

## Supportive supplements

| Supplement | Daily dosage | Good for ... |
|---|---|---|
| Zinc citrate or taurate | 50 milligrams | Balances mood and oestrogen production; helps maximise the use of magnesium in muscle relaxation |
| Vitamin B6 | 25 milligrams | Works with zinc to relieve mood swings and depression |
| 5-HTP | 150 milligrams | Supports serotonin production |
| Iron | 20 milligrams | Prevents anaemia; maintains energy |
| Omega-3 fish oil | 1 gram | Balances hormones; relieves uterine contractions |
| Omega-6 (starflower oil) | 500 milligrams | Reduces breast tenderness and lumpiness |

## MENSTRUATION

It has become the standard to prescribe teenage girls, some as young as 14, the oral contraceptive pill in order to 'regulate' their periods. It concerns me that this has become such a preoccupation for us. Puberty is tough, not only emotionally but also physically; the process of girls changing into young women has never been a smooth road. In health matters today we have a tendency to over-examine what is a fairly normal situation until it starts to look like a problem. Irregular or heavy periods in young girls are not necessarily things to worry about. Some girls won't be able to predict when their periods are due, and with others periods may be heavy or extremely sparse; others still may find them very painful. Every woman can relate to this. But the question is: 'When should we interfere?'

This is a very personal decision, and one that can only be made on an individual basis. If the problems are manageable, we should leave things alone and let nature take its course. If, however, a young woman has a number of menstrual irregularities, is taking days off school or bleeding very heavily, then something should certainly be done about it. But prescribing the pill seems a strange way to address these problems. It doesn't regulate anything; on the contrary, it suppresses ovarian function, supplements the body with artificial hormones, and then stops them every 21 days to allow a 'regular' hormonal withdrawal bleed. This is fine if the girl or young woman needs contraception; there is nothing more traumatic than an unwanted pregnancy. But if the girl concerned is not sexually active, then we should question whether this ought to be the method of choice. The pill only masks symptoms and doesn't solve the underlying problem at all. Often, too, young women's bodies are not yet mature enough to have had a chance to regulate their periods naturally.

Replenishing progesterone can certainly normalise problematic menstrual irregularities. Once again we are 'topping up' or balancing progesterone with a bio-identical hormone rather than suppressing our natural function with questionable synthetic hormones. Progesterone can also help regulate a woman's periods if she bleeds too often, too heavily and infrequently.

Many books have been written about progesterone and its benefits. The 'happy hormone' can have what seems like miraculous effects, but it's a *balanced* endocrine system that is truly miraculous.

## Adrienne's story

### ACNE AND POLYCYSTIC OVARY SYNDROME

**The Hormone Doctor:** Adrienne was a smart 28-year-old who came to me just after her engagement. She wanted to prepare herself for her forthcoming marriage and the life she had ahead of her. She had three major concerns: her health, her fertility and the problems she'd had in the past with acne.

At the age of 20 Adrienne had been diagnosed with polycystic ovary syndrome (PCOS) after her periods had completely stopped. PCOS affects about five per cent of all women. Women who have been diagnosed with polycystic ovaries are usually overweight, have infrequent periods and do not ovulate regularly, which may lead to infertility. They can also have excessive body hair and acne because they produce increased amounts of testosterone.

When she came to see me, Adrienne told me she had recently put on weight and had broken out in severe acne. She had been on the contraceptive pill for the last 11 years, and had no real idea what her cycle – or her skin – would be like without it.

We had a long discussion about all the things that would be necessary to achieve her goals – a healthy body, successful fertility and beautiful skin. I warned her that things might get a little worse before they got better. By this I meant that it was possible her skin problems would return and her periods might be either absent or irregular in the initial phase of the treatment, but Adrienne was very willing to take these risks. She was only too aware of the difficulties that women who suffer from PCOS have in falling pregnant. Of course, her self-consciousness played its role too; she did not want to be constantly breaking out in spots during her new life with her husband.

The first thing I advised her to do was to come off the pill to see how her cycle and skin would respond, and whether her general sense of wellbeing would alter. In my opinion there are two cases where the pill is over-prescribed – one is in the treatment of acne and the other in trying to regulate periods.

The second most important aspect of Adrienne's treatment was her nutrition. It is well documented that PCOS and acne can both respond favourably to proper nutrition. Adrienne was a wonderful patient who was motivated by and open to Vicki's and my advice. I asked her to come back to me two months after coming off the pill, and in the meantime I put her in Vicki's capable hands.

**The Nutritionist:** Adrienne had read a great deal about nutritional intervention in the cases of severe acne and PCOS, but had been confused by the contradictory information she'd come across. I had Adrienne keep a food diary and went through this with her in fine detail to determine where she could make changes.

I noticed that while in general Adrienne did not eat much fatty food, she seemed unable to resist cheese and ice-cream – foods she admitted being 'passionate' about – she had even invested in an ice-cream maker so she could make her own concoctions. She was aware that full-fat cream would contribute to her skin problems and had successfully developed half-fat ice-creams using egg yolks.

I told her that her use of the pill had protected her from the full effects of her eating habits. Now she was coming off the pill, she would have to cut out all dairy foods to prevent a major outbreak, since dairy is so high in saturated fats. I pointed out that the beauty of having her own ice-cream maker was that she could experiment with the rich tastes and textures of almond- and cashew-nut milks instead of dairy. I also suggested a range of dips, spreads and sauces that she could try in place of cheese.

Already a good cook, Adrienne was enthusiastic about taking a new approach. Fortunately for her, chocolate had never been one of her passions, and she considered it very much a 'take it or leave it' food, so I told her to leave it out altogether. Those who aren't passionate chocoholics usually turn to cheap, commercial chocolate when they do eat chocolate at all, and it's this stuff that is packed with the dairy solids and sugars that contribute to acne. If Adrienne had really loved her chocolate, I would have advised she eat small amounts of dark, low-sugar chocolate high in cocoa solids.

I have worked with many women with both acne and PCOS who are seeking a more natural solution than using synthetic hormones or long-term courses of antibiotics to 'mask' the symptoms. Of my PCOS clients looking to improve their fertility, the ones who have gone on to give birth were those who cut animal dairy produce from their diet. People have speculated about a link between the consumption of cow's dairy produce and PCOS (see Colette Harris and Dr Adam Carey's book, *PCOS: A Woman's Guide to Dealing with Polycystic Ovary Syndrome*). While Australian farmers do not follow the practice of including growth hormones in their cattle feed, this is sadly not the case throughout the countries of the EU. Such growth hormones, even in minute quantities, may alter the balance of oestrogens and progesterone in susceptible women, thus creating the environment for PCOS to proliferate. And the saturated-fat content of milk, cream, butter and cheese is likely to aggravate even the slightest case of acne.

**The Hormone Doctor:** After being off the pill for two months, Adrienne came back for her follow-up consultation. She was looking brighter and feeling more energetic, but was very disappointed that her periods hadn't returned and that her skin had deteriorated, despite her following Vicki's recommendations to the letter. I asked her to be patient and explained that we wanted her body to find its own rhythm and balance. She'd had 11 years of suppressed ovarian function – they'd need a bit of time to be woken up. I told her that I might recommend progesterone treatment if her periods had not returned after six months. I also asked that she have an ultrasound of her ovaries to see if any cysts had returned.

Adrienne came back after another two months; her periods had still not restarted, and the ultrasound did not confirm polycystic ovaries but was merely suggestive of PCOS. Adrienne was a perfect patient, but now she was beginning to get anxious about whether her periods would ever return. I suggested that she carry out a monthly female-hormone profile saliva test so that we could closely monitor her hormones.

The results of these saliva tests showed normal oestradiol and testosterone levels but continuously low progesterone levels. I then decided to treat Adrienne with cyclical progesterone cream – two weeks on and two weeks off. This had a practically immediate effect, and she had her first period four weeks later.

Adrienne's wedding date was fast approaching and her skin had improved, although she was still getting the occasional spot. She said she was feeling more confident, and wasn't as concerned about her skin now that she was seeing slow but continuous improvement.

I saw Adrienne again after her wedding. Her periods were occurring at six-to-eight-weekly intervals. She was thrilled about this and was very keen to get pregnant as soon as possible. Her whole demeanour had improved – she was intensely happy and in love. We decided to leave things be. The only thing I advised her to do at this stage was take prenatal vitamins.

Adrienne continued with the progesterone treatment and kept following Vicki's nutritional advice. Six months later she came to visit me again – this time for a blood test to confirm her pregnancy. The tests were positive and I referred her to an obstetrician for further care.

Adrienne's periods returned six months after the birth of her child and she has had regular periods ever since. Her skin cleared up during the pregnancy and has remained clear to this day. She went on to have a second child and had no problems conceiving.

**The Nutritionist:** Adrienne continued the dairy-free approach beyond her first pregnancy, realising that the advantages were broader than simply affecting her skin and hormone balance. In fact, not only has her husband adopted the diet, but her two children have been raised dairy-free and have not had cradle cap or eczema in infancy, nor any ear, nose or throat problems, all of which has been linked with the consumption of cow's dairy foods. Neither have they had any issues with sinusitis, rhinitis or food intolerances. This is a perfect example of how staying on a dedicated integrative health plan can reap long-term rewards.

## Acne and PCOS – foods to avoid

These foods should be off your list if you suffer from acne and PCOS:

- all dairy products
- caffeine – particularly coffee
- refined sugars
- saturated fat found in fatty red meat, bacon, sausages

- alcohol
- fried foods (both deep- and shallow-fried)

## Acne and PCOS megafoods

Make sure you stock up on these megafoods to help combat acne and PCOS:

- zinc-rich foods – shellfish, chicken, turkey, eggs and lean red meat; soy beans, chick peas, lentils and split peas for vegetarians
- omega-3, -6 and -9-rich seeds – flaxseeds, sunflower and pumpkin seeds
- diindolemethane (DIM)-rich foods – cauliflower, broccoli, Brussels sprouts and cabbages
- vitamin C – kiwifruit, sweet potatoes, capsicum (bell peppers), watercress and broccoli
- vitamin E – avocado, wheat-germ extract, Brazil nuts, pumpkin-seed oil and oily fish
- alpha- and beta-carotenes – capsicum (bell peppers), squashes, pumpkin, carrots, cantaloupe melon, tomatoes, mango and papaya
- chromium-rich foods – shellfish, Brewer's yeast (from the health-food shop – sprinkle it on porridge), whole-wheat products and baked beans (organic, sugar-free varieties)

You should also take the supportive supplements listed in the table on the next page; they can be beneficial for both acne and PCOS.

It is vital to balance blood sugar levels to regulate insulin-release from the pancreas. An excess of insulin may be associated with polycystic ovaries, obesity and menstrual irregularities. Eat little and often, combining some protein with every meal to maintain balanced levels of blood sugar.

## Supportive supplements

| Supplement | Daily dosage | Good for . . . |
|---|---|---|
| Zinc citrate | 50 micrograms at night | Helps heal and repair scarring, and assists in the production of insulin for those with PCOS |
| Vitamin C | 1 milligram twice daily | Supports collagen production and skin repair |
| Vitamin E | 400 micrograms | Increases skin tone, elasticity and hydration |
| Vitamin A | 2500 IUs | Repairs skin and helps balance hormones |
| Diindolemethane (DIM) | 100 milligrams | Promotes natural oestrogen metabolism |
| Flaxseed oil | 2–4 tablespoons | Reduces inflammation associated with acne and helps balance female hormones in those with PCOS |
| Chromium picolinate | 25 micrograms | Supports a balanced production of insulin, which is often excessive in those with PCOS |

# 5

# all about testosterone

## THE HORMONE ALL WOMEN NEED

Yes, that's right, women need testosterone. We produce testosterone in our ovaries (and a little bit in our adrenal glands). It's common to think that testosterone is a male hormone, but it is also a vital hormone for women. The difference is that women need much less of it than men. It has multiple qualities for both sexes: it increases sexual desire; it gives you a sense of wellbeing, confidence and assertiveness; it helps you withstand stress and provides energy; it can strengthen your bone and increase muscle tone and muscle mass; it can relieve joint and muscle pain and can also decrease cholesterol levels.

Women come to see me for many reasons, but the majority of them come because of their menopausal symptoms, which we know can vary widely, as everyone experiences their 'own' menopause. The most common complaint women have – even more common than hot flushes – is low libido. I would say that 85 per cent of my patients complain of low sex drive, and these were patients across the board, of all ages. It is not unusual for me to see patients in their 30s, 40s, 50s all on the same day and all complaining of the same symptom – low libido. Why does this happen?

# WHEN YOU'D RATHER GO TO BED WITH A NICE CUP OF TEA

Some of my patients are initially quite shy to talk about their sexual relationships. Many feel guilty that they love their partners but do not desire them physically. Others pretend to enjoy sex to keep their husbands happy. For some it is more of a chore or a duty; it feels more of an effort than a pleasure. Many of my patients say that if it were not for their partners, they would never need to have sex again – it is the thing furthest from their mind. And then again, a large group of patients complain that they have lost their sex drive and want it back. Women who have enjoyed sex and been very active previously can't understand what has happened to them and their libido.

During my 15 years in women's health, I have become an unintentional sex therapist for many women. Everything we read in women's magazines and see in films about romantic love and passionate sex is just not happening in the real world. Where has the sex drive of so many women (and some men) gone? Isn't love synonymous with having a healthy sex life? Why does it decrease for so many after marriage and practically extinguish itself when they reach their 50s?

Lifestyle, stress, family, children, hormones – these can all play a role. For some it is a combination of these factors.

## Beatrice's story

### 'TOO TIRED, TOO EXHAUSTED, TOO BUSY TO HAVE SEX'

**The Hormone Doctor:** Beatrice was in her 30s and married to a high-flying private-equity trader. She had stopped having intercourse with her husband after the birth of their second child – and that was six years ago! She didn't miss sex and apparently neither did her husband (but he was not my patient so I don't know why). She was concerned that she had lost all sexual desire and didn't quite understand what was happening. She was mildly depressed, excessively tired and lacked stamina. She came to me because she thought it might have been a hormonal problem.

After talking for some time with Beatrice, I realised that there was no intimacy between her and her husband and that she essentially lived the life of a single mother (albeit with far greater financial security and more creature comforts than the average single mum). Beatrice's husband spent 12 or more hours a day at work and perhaps only two or three at home. He usually only had any relationship with the children and his wife on weekends. His focus was his career.

With a workaholic partner and no intimacy in their relationship, it was no wonder Beatrice had lost her desire for sex with her husband. She did want to resume a sexual relationship with him, but after six years was too scared to approach him let alone seduce him.

All Beatrice's blood tests for various hormone levels came back normal but in a low range. Of course, I could have given her some testosterone supplementation, which might have helped her to be more assertive and confident and might have countered her depression. Instead, however, I advised her to see a marriage counsellor so that she could begin to address the problems in her relationship. Until now, she and her husband were simply practising 'avoidance therapy'. From the outside, Beatrice's family life looked okay, but from the inside both partners were becoming increasingly introverted and lonely. 'Hormones' were not the cause. Testosterone (for both partners) might have helped, but in this case any hormonal treatment had to wait, since the relationship needed to be sorted out first.

When Beatrice returned to my clinic a couple of months later, she reported that she and her husband had been to marriage counselling and that it was helping. They had resumed a sexual relationship but Beatrice admitted it was not particularly gratifying for her. She confided to me that she had never experienced an orgasm nor had she ever masturbated. (It is times like these I become an accidental sex therapist.) I prescribed for Beatrice a testosterone cream to be applied daily to her clitoris and around the vagina. The intention was that it would increase sensitivity so that with stimulation she could achieve an orgasm.

Beatrice and her husband both wanted a successful marriage and family life, and after beginning to address their problems were on the way to achieving these aims.

## Margaret and John's story

### INABILITY TO HAVE SEX

**The Hormone Doctor:** Margaret and John were a lovely couple. They were both in their mid-60s and for both this was their second marriage. Margaret was a widow and John had been divorced. Both had grown-up children and were retired; they enjoyed travelling and wanted to enjoy their retirement together. They had been married for 10 years and were extremely happy as a couple except for the fact that they could not have intercourse. The entrance to Margaret's vagina (the introitus) had become too small and tight, so that penetration was impossible.

I explained to Margaret and John how important hormones – both oestrogen and testosterone – were for the vaginal tissues. Margaret had stopped her conventional HRT approximately five years earlier, but was happy to start bio-identical hormone therapy, especially as it would be tailored to her needs. I prescribed her a lozenge with oestradiol and progesterone, along with Vagifem vaginal tablets and a testosterone cream to apply on the outside of her genitalia, including the clitoris. Vagifem would help the tissues of the vagina and testosterone would strengthen the tissue of the introitus and labia.

After starting the treatment, Margaret noticed that slowly but surely her vagina was becoming plumper, better lubricated and less fragile. Both Margaret and John were patient; they took their time and were gentle. After six months of treatment, Margaret's vagina was elastic and strong enough to enable them to have proper intercourse. After that Margaret needed to use the Vagifem and testosterone only intermittently, when she felt that they were required, but she stayed on her daily oestradiol and progesterone lozenge.

**The Nutritionist:** Nutrition plays a part in keeping both our external and internal 'skins' properly hydrated and lubricated. And the answer isn't simply to drink plenty of water.

Every skin cell in your body is made up of collagen, fibrinogen and essential fatty acids. In order for skin cells to be regenerated, they need ample hydration on the outer layers of skin, and essential fats to allow the reconstruction and rebuilding of new layers of skin. In other words, to have soft, plump, healthy skin, including that found in the genital area, you must eat plenty of foods rich in essential fatty acids.

To ensure that you are getting enough of the wonderful nutrients needed for good skin, include plenty of the following in your regular regime.

## Skin-plumping megafoods

- sunflower seeds, pumpkin seeds, sesame seeds and nut butters (for example, cashew and almond)

- olive, flaxseed, pumpkin-seed, avocado and walnut oils – all are rich sources of omega-3 and -6 essential fatty acids, and make delicious alternatives to salad dressings
- avocados – they have an abundance of vitamin E, which is important for skin elasticity and suppleness
- kiwifruit, sweet potatoes, spinach and citrus fruits – all are rich in vitamin C, which helps to produce collagen; our bodies cannot store this vital vitamin so include daily helpings of these foods in your diet

## Gerry's story

### INABILITY TO ORGASM: 'IS IT MY FAULT?'

**The Hormone Doctor:** This was another case where I became an accidental sex therapist.

Gerry was 38 years old, married, had regular sex with her husband but had never had an orgasm. She didn't know what 'all the fuss was about'. She came to me because she thought that she might be lacking testosterone and wanted to know if it was 'her fault'.

Of course, it takes two to tango, and a woman has to tell her partner what she likes and what pleases her if she is going to enjoy sex. If she doesn't know what pleases her, however, it can be even more difficult for her partner. Gerry never masturbated because when she tried she said that she never 'felt anything'. She was one of my many patients who said that they did not have a strong sex drive, although this did not preclude her from being able to achieve an orgasm. I decided to prescribe Gerry a low-dose testosterone cream to apply to her pubic area and her clitoris.

Just a couple of days after she began using the testosterone cream, Gerry started having sexual dreams for the first time in her life. She noticed that her clitoris started becoming more sensitive and she started feeling less inhibited with her husband. She told him that she was using testosterone cream and that she was feeling 'sexier'.

When she came back for a review and a repeat prescription, she told me that she was enjoying sex much more and regularly achieving an orgasm.

**The Nutritionist:** Marion and I have heard countless similar stories in both our clinics. It saddens me to think that some women have never experienced an orgasm and don't know that anything can be done to help.

Whenever I suspect that a client might have low sensitivity for any type of taste, touch or smell, I always test their zinc levels. Zinc is such an important nutrient for the senses.

One of the richest sources of zinc is oysters, which is why they are commonly referred to as an aphrodisiac (actually, all shellfish contain zinc). Likewise caviar is rich in zinc. Other good sources include pine nuts, spinach, rye, almonds and sesame seeds, as well as whole grains, particularly brown rice.

## DECLINING TESTOSTERONE AT PERI-MENOPAUSE

Most of my patients who complain of low libido are peri-menopausal. By definition this means they are around the time of menopause, when their periods are becoming irregular but have not totally ceased. Their ovaries are beginning to produce less hormone than before, with fluctuating levels from day to day. Nothing is either consistent or dependable any more – their menstruation, energy, moods and libido are all in a state of flux. Low libido is the result of hormonal imbalance or hormonal fluctuation – everything is on the move but more often on the way down than up. This is one of the reasons that so many women complain of a low sex drive when they reach the peri-menopausal stage.

Here is one of my favourite stories about libido and testosterone, even though this was one time when I really could not help my patient.

## *Anni's story*

### LOW LIBIDO: 'CAN YOU FIX ME?'

**The Hormone Doctor:** Anni came to my surgery saying that her husband had sent her to see me so that I could 'fix' her. He had come to one of my public talks and thought that I would be the person to help her with her low libido.

Anni told me that she loved her husband dearly. She had got married when she was 20 and her husband was 22 years older. They had been married for 26 years; she had borne him three children, the youngest of whom was 10, and she had been through thick and thin with him. He was an extremely successful businessman, still very attractive and charming, but she no longer desired him sexually. She told me that her husband was her best friend but she didn't want him as a lover any more. Of course he objected to this and he thought that if I prescribed Anni some testosterone all would be well again.

Well, it wasn't going to be that easy. Anni continued to tell me that she had a very strong libido and in fact was having the best sex of her life. Anni had two lovers, one who was very much in love with her and wanted her to leave her husband and the other a friend with whom she'd had a casual relationship for the past three years.

Anni knew she was in dangerous territory, but she said she was having 'too much fun' and wasn't ready to stop yet. One thing was certain: she loved her husband and her family and did not want to lose them. But she also knew she was behaving like an extremely naughty child.

Anni's husband must have been disappointed I couldn't 'fix' her. Far from it. Anni needed to face some realities about her relationship and make some big decisions. But Anni wasn't ready for counselling. I do hope that she has sorted things out now.

## TESTOSTERONE IN THE FIGHT AGAINST OSTEOPOROSIS

There are so many reasons women need testosterone. One big one is that testosterone is an anabolic steroid. Yes, I know this sounds like scary bodybuilder stuff – huge abs, bulging muscles in tight T-shirts, hairy legs and a deep voice. And no, if you take testosterone supplementation you won't grow a beard or need a bikini wax down to your knees, I promise.

The fact that testosterone is a steroid means that it is capable of building tissue. Testosterone can build muscle, increase tone and reduce fat deposits in the body. And the best news of all is that it can build bone. We are all frightened of developing osteoporosis, or brittle bones, as we age, and testosterone is an important hormone in fighting this disease that affects so many women.

# HORMONES AS 'ANTI-AGEING' MEDICINE?

I am not crazy about the term 'anti-ageing', which is used by some in the medical profession and in the media when talking about bio-identical hormone therapy. Hormone therapy isn't about cheating fate or achieving some amazing 'look' well into your 50s and 60s. The unavoidable reality is that we all age. The real question is *how* we age.

Assuring a good hormone balance is all about maintaining your health, your bones, your quality of life, and securing an active and hopefully disease-free time long after you have retired. If you feel well there will be an aura of vitality and health around you. You look and feel beautiful when you are healthy. No amount of plastic surgery, Botox or other 'anti-ageing' procedures will make you feel this way. They can't strengthen your bones, ease your aching joints or increase your energy levels.

If someone asked me to give just one reason why many women should be on bio-identical hormone therapy, I would say for their bones. Testosterone, in combination with oestrogen and progesterone, is the best protection any woman can have for her bones. Oestrogen maintains bone tissue, progesterone builds bone tissue and testosterone strengthens bone tissue. I think this a dream combination for any woman who has a low bone density, a family history of osteoporosis or who has gone into an early menopause.

I ask most of my peri-menopausal patients to have a bone-density scan. It is important that they know how healthy their bones are and that together we monitor them over time. After all, I practise preventative medicine – my interest lies in keeping my patients healthy and strengthening their constitution as necessary.

Low bone density, or osteopaenia, is unfortunately very common – it is considered normal for women over 50 to have a low bone density. So what are we expected to do about it? Wait around while our bone health declines? Take a bit of extra calcium and then, when the first fracture occurs and we are diagnosed with osteoporosis, start with the heavy pharmaceutical drugs? We want to *prevent* osteoporosis.

Exercise and diet play a huge role in the prevention of osteoporosis. But in addition to these twin weapons, supplementation of oestrogen, progesterone and testosterone can give women the best defence possible. As I've seen time and time again in my clinic, a healthy balance of these hormones not only prevents the onset of osteoporosis, it can significantly reverse bone-density decline so that a woman can regain normal bone strength. I have seen countless patients – too many to give examples here – whose bone density has improved significantly after bio-identical hormone therapy with these three hormones in combination. Some came with osteoporosis and others with osteopaenia. Most could attain a normal bone density after two to three years of treatment, and they could maintain it if they kept up their treatment regime, exercise and appropriate nutrition. These results are much better than these patients could have expected from conventional medication for the treatment of osteoporosis.

## NUTRITION FOR BONE HEALTH

How many times has your doctor insisted on giving you calcium to 'protect' your bones? And how many times have you had to go back with nothing more to show for the treatment than constipation? If it hasn't happened to you, it will have certainly have happened to someone you know. The problems occur because many GPs do not prescribe calcium in conjunction with magnesium. Calcium cannot be absorbed into the bone tissue without a certain amount of magnesium in your body.

And to maintain bone strength you also need vitamin D3, manganese and boron – there are many complex supplements on the market that can provide all these nutrients, along with two other much-needed nutrients, methylsulfonylmethane (MSM) and chondroitin.

## Supportive supplements

When looking for an optimal bone-supporting complex, make sure it contains the following nutrients.

| Nutrient | Amount |
|---|---|
| Magnesium and calcium | In a 2:1 ratio (for example, 600 milligrams : 300 milligrams) |
| Silica | 55 micrograms |
| Boron | 0.25 milligrams |
| Manganese | 1.5 milligrams |
| Vitamin D3 (or cholecalciferol) | 600 IUs |

*Did you know . . . ?*

Even if you live in a sunny part of the world, it's a good idea to take a nutritional supplement of vitamin D to support bone health. Nowadays most people use high-protection sunscreens and wear sunglasses that shield the retina of the eye from the harmful effects of UV light. The downside is that this can prevent sunlight activating the production of vitamin D in the body.

And now to the bone-building megafoods. Do you drink milk and eat cheese to up your calcium intake and help your bones? If so, consider this: there is virtually no magnesium in dairy produce, which means that unless you are eating lots of green vegetables, you're probably not absorbing the calcium.

There is actually more calcium in a head of broccoli than in half a litre of milk, and the broccoli has the added benefit of containing plenty of magnesium – it's the perfect bone food! So too are celery, asparagus and cauliflower.

## Bone-building megafoods

- broccoli, asparagus, celery, cauliflower
- all nuts and seeds, tahini, cashew- and almond-nut butters
- sardines, anchovies and pilchards (include their tiny bones to get their best nutrients)
- spinach, kale, Savoy cabbage
- calf and chicken livers, egg yolks
- lentils, split peas, rye, buckwheat (also contains rutin, which strengthens the small capillaries throughout the body – a preventative for thread veins)
- green leafy vegetables
- whole grains
- sea vegetables, in particular kelp
- onions

## Mineral-robbing foods to avoid

- caffeine
- alcohol
- refined sugars and sweeteners
- margarine

## Bruna's story

### BATTLING OSTEOPOROSIS AND AN EATING DISORDER

**The Hormone Doctor:** Bruna was 57 years old and had a history of osteoporosis when she first came to my clinic. As soon as she walked in the door it was clear to me that she most likely had a history of anorexia too, a fact she confirmed during the consultation.

Bruna was 168 centimetres (5 feet 6 inches) tall and weighed just 49 kilograms (7½ stone; 108 pounds). She was a very intelligent woman, was director of her own company, and had a 23-year-old daughter. She was very concerned about her appearance and realised that her eating disorder had contributed to her severe osteoporosis. She had been taking Fosamax (a drug that helps improve bone density) for the previous four years, which had maintained but not improved her bone density, and she was still osteoporotic. In other words, the Fosamax had stopped the decline but had not caused a significant increase in her bone density.

One of Bruna's main symptoms was a lack of energy and concentration, which she found frustrating, being a perfectionist in her professional and private life.

As usual, I asked Bruna to bring along copies of each of the bone-density tests she'd had. I carried out blood tests, which confirmed not only that she was in the menopause, but also that she had a mildly under-functioning thyroid. With her history, I was surprised that she was not on conventional HRT, but I found out that her obsession with her weight had made her very reluctant to take conventional HRT for fear of gaining weight.

Bruna was well aware of her eating disorder and had learned to manage her life around it. Besides her osteoporosis, she had no other symptoms or signs of nutritional deficiencies. I told her that she needed hormone supplementation in the form of low-dose armour thyroid (a standardised dose of T3 and T4 – see page 178), and also a combination of oestrogen, progesterone and testosterone to build up her bone density. Of course, I had to reassure her that there was no risk of weight gain providing the prescription was suitably balanced for her. I pointed out that I would monitor this carefully with regular blood tests and yearly bone-density tests.

Bruna was already under the care of an endocrinologist to monitor her bone density, and was always cautious to ensure that all her specialists were informed of her increased care and prescriptions.

I saw Bruna six weeks after her initial consultation, and she commented on how much her energy levels had already improved, and that she was also sleeping better. After three months, her blood tests confirmed that there was an improvement in her thyroid function.

We repeated a bone-density scan after 12 months of treatment and Bruna was thrilled to see that there was a significant increase in her bone density. She was still in the osteoporotic range, but was heading away from danger.

Initially, her endocrinologist was sceptical about Bruna's use of bio-identical hormones, but at the same time he did not dissuade her from taking them. After two years of treatment, he agreed it was doing her good, which she found very reassuring.

Bruna now no longer needs to fear a possible fracture if she trips over, and her energy levels and cognitive function have improved tremendously. On the whole, she has become a healthier, happier and stronger woman.

Since Bruna was always obsessed about her diet and weight, I referred her to Vicki, who has treated more than a hundred patients suffering from eating disorders such as anorexia, bulimia and binge-eating habits.

**The Nutritionist:** Bruna stunned me on two levels. First in a positive way, in that she was so beautiful. And secondly in a negative way, in that she was overly disciplined about her intake of certain foods, preferring – without exception – healthy and organic foods. This condition of being obsessive about the origins and derivations of certain foods to the point of being extremely restrictive is now commonly termed orthorexia and is sometimes found in women (and a small number of men) who have been anorexic for a number of years.

Despite being very slender, Bruna was definitely not emaciated. We concentrated on which foods Bruna should include in her diet on a regular basis to support her bone health.

It's a common misconception that calcium is the most important nutrient for supporting bone health. This is only part of the story – calcium cannot be absorbed into the bone matrix without the inclusion of magnesium, and many women, especially those who work in stressful situations, are magnesium-deficient because their adrenal glands use up magnesium in managing stress.

In an effort to avoid starchy foods, Bruna ate very few whole grains, which are the richest source of magnesium. I could not persuade her to include whole grains in her diet because she was worried they would cause bloating and weight gain, so I insisted that she instead eat plenty of dark green vegetables, such as watercress, rocket, parsley, kale and Savoy cabbage, as well as almonds (soaked so that they were more easily digestible), to ensure she got plenty of magnesium on a daily basis. I also suggested that she eat high-protein foods such as sardines, mackerel and herrings regularly for lunch, and include sesame seed paste (tahini) as a dip for salad vegetables in the mid-afternoon. These are all rich sources of calcium as alternatives to dairy, which Bruna had cut out of her diet years before.

Bruna's low-fat diet meant that nuts were usually off the menu, but when I pointed out that she needed only a small palmful of almonds, hazelnuts, pecans or walnuts daily to provide a good source of calcium, boron and manganese, she agreed that she would include these and think of them as her 'bone builders'.

Marion had tested Bruna's vitamin D status, which was deficient. Vitamin D is essential for bone health, and Bruna always looked very pale, having actively avoided the sun in order to protect her appearance. Vitamin D is activated in the body in the presence of sunlight, so Marion had suggested that Bruna always wear a sunscreen with a high sun-protection factor but ensure that she removed her sunglasses for at least 15 minutes a day to allow the sun to stimulate the vitamin D through her retinas.

I further suggested that she take a supplement of kelp, one of the best natural sources of vitamin D, and to add onions to her salads as another source of vitamin D. Finally, I gave her a bone-supporting multi-mineral supplement, including magnesium, calcium, manganese, boron, silica and vitamin D3.

Bruna was thankful to understand which nutrients worked in synergy to support bone health, and took on my food recommendations. She realised that her diet had been overly limited and was pleased to be able to overcome certain 'food fears'. There is no doubt that her positive bone-density test performed a year later was attributable to all three forms of treatment: bio-identical hormone supplementation, an increase in the variety of foods in her diet, and nutritional supplements. This is a perfect example of how all three approaches can combine to produce a great result that each on its own could not have achieved.

## THE OTHER GREAT THINGS ABOUT TESTOSTERONE

Testosterone has even more beneficial qualities than just increasing your bone density and libido. It can also make you more assertive, alert and confident, and give you a sense of vitality. Many of my patients complain of fatigue, aching joints and a lack of motivation. They feel flat or melancholy, are indecisive and lack stamina. Testosterone-deficient patients also complain that they feel flabby, that they have lost muscle tone and that their armpit and pubic hair has thinned. These are quite common symptoms of testosterone deficiency.

It is wonderful to experience how a little testosterone supplementation can change everything for the better.

## Bettina's story

### LACKING STAMINA: 'I CAN'T FACE THE DAY'

**The Hormone Doctor:** Bettina was a school teacher. She was 45, peri-menopausal, had been on progesterone cream for a year and was feeling much better for it. When she came to me for a review and repeat prescription, she complained of her fatigue and how she woke up in the morning wanting to face neither the day nor her Year 12 pupils. She said she wasn't depressed but felt she didn't have the strength to manage her students and was losing control in the classroom. Until now this had never been a problem – she had always commanded their respect and felt very confident in her role as a teacher.

I checked Bettina's thyroid levels because an under-functioning thyroid can produce the sorts of symptoms she talked about. While we were at it, we tested her testosterone levels. It turned out Bettina's thyroid was fine but her testosterone levels were low.

I added 2 milligrams per day of testosterone in a cream to Bettina's bio-identical hormone therapy regime. I told her of the possible side effects if I had prescribed her too much, and that it might make her a bit aggressive and irritable. She didn't mind this. She said that a bit of aggression would be a good thing in her situation!

I saw Bettina again two months later and she said she was feeling great and now had lots of energy. 'I feel like a teenager again,' she said. 'And look, I'm even getting some pimples!' Oops, well, obviously I had given her a bit too much, because high testosterone levels can also cause oily skin, acne and loss of hair on the head. I reduced the dosage by half and Bettina was pleased to have all the benefits of feeling well again with plenty of assertiveness, but this time without the pimples.

---

### Did you know . . . ?

Exercise increases testosterone levels naturally, and testosterone increases your energy. In turn, this can help to make you more assertive, more motivated and more 'in control'. In other words, you become physically and emotionally strong. Knowing all this, why would you *not* exercise? It's such a great solution, and so beneficial in many more ways. Increased heart health, bone health, muscle strength and tone, as well as weight management and a more youthful figure are all advantages of regular exercise and its concomitant increased testosterone levels.

---

Testosterone makes us sexier and stronger and, in many ways, more feminine because it gives us the confidence to be the person we are. Stella is a fine example of this.

## Stella's story

### SUDDEN LOSS OF SEX DRIVE: 'IT'S JUST NOT ME'

**The Nutritionist:** Stella is a favourite client of mine whom I have been seeing in my clinic for a number of years. She is successful in her product-design and corporate-branding business, wonderfully elegant and, without a doubt, one of the smartest women I have ever met.

She had come to see me for a number of minor complaints over the years, but more recently she had been concerned about her noticeable lack of interest in sex with her partner. Stella has a long-term partner with whom she is very close, respecting his amicable relationship with his ex-wife and mother of his children without any of the jealousy and insecurity that other women in that situation can often display. She had always had a strong sex drive, claiming she was 'more like a man in her sexual appetite than a woman'.

For Stella, to find herself without any sex drive was more than a little disturbing. Her hormonal profile indicated that she had entered the menopause over the last 18 months. She'd had no periods for more than 20 months, and showed lowered oestrogen levels and virtually no progesterone or testosterone. Yet there was almost no change to Stella's appearance, energy levels or self-esteem. The only noticeable change was that Stella simply didn't want sex any more; in fact, she didn't even want intimate contact of any kind. This understandably upset her partner.

I suggested that Stella see Marion to have her hormone levels restored. Clearly it was her lowered oestrogen, progesterone and testosterone in particular that were responsible for her loss of sex drive.

**The Hormone Doctor:** When Stella came to see me, she reiterated that she had no complaints other than a disturbingly non-existent sex drive. She felt she just wasn't her 'old self' any more. She hoped that testosterone supplementation would do the trick.

I explained that I don't treat symptoms, I treat the whole person and that she was lacking all three hormones: oestrogen, progesterone and testosterone. I was concerned not only with Stella's loss of libido, but also with maintaining her bone health, the integrity of her skin and her brain health. Working actively to redress her hormone deficiencies would mean she could maintain her health and vitality rather than just wait for symptoms to arise.

I prescribed a combination of oestrogen, progesterone and testosterone in a cream that Stella was to apply daily after her shower. If she were to come back to me still complaining of a low sex drive, I could also prescribe a higher dose testosterone cream for application to her genital area to increase its sensitivity.

**The Nutritionist:** At the same time as Marion was treating Stella, I recommended a supplement for her that includes maca – a Peruvian plant-derived herbal supplement that is well known for its testosterone-enhancing properties and for improving sex drive. (Note that maca should not be taken by women who have a history of breast cancer or who are currently undergoing chemotherapy.)

Finally, I gave Stella a concentrated blue-green algae powder to include in her breakfast smoothie every morning. There is no other known food source on the planet that is as nutrient-dense as blue-green algae and, as absorption of nutrients decreases with age, I consider it to be one of the most important food supplements a woman can take to increase her general vitality.

Stella started to respond to this combination of hormones and supplements within eight to 10 weeks. She and her partner decided to go away for a honeymoon-style weekend to a favourite place where they had spent one of their first weekends together. Stella said she found herself 're-attracted' to her man, with no extra effort or forced amour required. She admitted to feeling almost sex-kittenish as she pranced out of the hotel bathroom wearing beautiful underwear. It was the start of a 'whole new chapter', as she described it, in their relationship, and she was enormously grateful for the 'rescue package' that had prevented a decline in an otherwise wonderful partnership.

# 6
# all about
# thyroid hormone

## THE HORMONE THAT KEEPS US SANE AND ENERGETIC

When I was a student at medical school (many moons ago), one of my lecturers in psychiatry told us always to consider a commonly occurring diagnosis before a rare one. He said that many, many people landed in psychiatric units severely depressed and at times suicidal or paranoid, but that these people did not have psychiatric disorders. Their symptoms were certainly considered psychiatric, but their cause wasn't. Of course, we pricked up our ears during what was usually a laborious lecture. Were people really being sent to psychiatric units when they weren't 'mad' at all? Why were they being sent there? Was there a conspiracy? This was starting to sound like a detective novel. My imagination ran wild and that particular lecture remains a memorable one for me.

Our lecturer was telling us that patients were being admitted into psychiatric units after trying antidepressants without success because no one had checked their thyroid hormone function. That's right, thyroid hormone doesn't just regulate your metabolism. Sure, it can make you fat or slim, slow you down or make you feel racy, but it is much more powerful than that.

Nearly 30 years after that lecture, I am still encountering what our professor warned us about. Many doctors don't consider Hypothyroidism, or under-functioning thyroid, first off when a patient presents with depression. It is not unusual to be offered antidepressants practically immediately when you complain of tiredness, not coping with your life and feeling depressed. In fact, hypothyroidism is becoming one of the most commonly missed diagnoses and yet its incidence is increasingly widespread.

## Jennifer's story

### DESPERATE AND NOWHERE TO GO!

**The Hormone Doctor:** Jennifer had a friend with her the first time I saw her. It was her friend who had heard about me, convinced Jennifer to come and even paid for the consultation. Jennifer could never have made it alone. She was desperate – really desperate. She was constantly exhausted but unable to sleep, and had reached a point where she thought life wasn't worth living. I heard how she had considered driving into a tree, but then baulked because she decided she could not inflict something like that on her family. She suffered bursts of anger and had nearly attacked her husband with a knife. She was at the end of her tether.

Jennifer had gone to both her GP and gynaecologist on various occasions, asking them to check her hormones, thinking that they could be the source of her trouble. Instead of getting the help she needed, Jennifer was reprimanded: she was told to pull herself together, that she had a family to take care of. She was prescribed antidepressants and anti-anxiety medication, and referred to a psychiatrist, with whom she had not yet made an appointment. She took the drugs but stopped shortly afterwards because she said they only made her feel worse. Her husband had taken over most of the daily chores and luckily her sons were in boarding school, because Jennifer didn't want them to see her in such a state. She had been feeling like this on and off for almost six months.

I certainly thought that the cause might be a severe case of fluctuating hormones. Jennifer was 47 and still had regular heavy periods. I thought she might also be anaemic, which could have contributed to her fatigue. I ran a series of blood tests, including a thyroid-function test, to see if they would confirm my hunches.

Jennifer's problem was hormonal, as she had suspected, and the problems lay with her thyroid. Her thyroid-stimulating hormone (TSH) was elevated. The normal range lies between 0.75 and 4.5, but Jennifer had a TSH of 37! (It's easy to get confused here: when a stimulating hormone is elevated, it means that the target organ is under-functioning.) Her thyroid gland was seriously under-functioning.

We discovered that Jennifer had Hashimoto's disease, one of the most common forms of underactive thyroid. Hashimoto's disease is often misdiagnosed as bipolar disorder and, less frequently, as anxiety disorder, but testing for anti-thyroid antibodies can resolve any diagnostic difficulty. People with this condition have elevated numbers of antibodies that attack their own thyroid. No wonder Jennifer was feeling so awful – she had a severe, longstanding under-functioning thyroid. If left untreated, Hashimoto's disease can lead to the debilitating thyroid psychosis, also known as 'myxoedema madness'. Not everyone with an under-functioning thyroid will suffer such extreme symptoms; this is just an example of how bad and 'mad' it can get.

I referred Jennifer to an endocrinologist for further evaluation, to make sure that I hadn't missed anything. She didn't need a psychiatrist. She had 'felt' what was wrong with her but been ignored by her doctors. This is a great pity, because it could have saved her many months of hell.

Had her friend not brought her to see me, she would have waited even longer for the right diagnosis.

The endocrinologist initially treated Jennifer with 50 micrograms of thyroxine daily then slowly increased the dosage to 100 micrograms. Her stamina returned and she was less depressed, but she was still severely traumatised by her six months of feeling 'mad' and out of control. She then saw a psychotherapist and underwent some cognitive behavioural therapy to manage her anxiety.

Jennifer is now more resilient, her confidence has returned and she is leading a 'normal' life again. Jennifer's was, of course, a very severe case of hypothyroidism but could so easily have been solved much earlier with straightforward blood tests.

*Did you know . . . ?*

The most severe case of hypothyroidism is called cretinism, where someone is born without a functioning thyroid gland. If not treated, the result is severely stunted mental and physical growth. These days, however, all newborn babies are screened for the condition; when picked up, cretinism can be treated with thyroxine and the child's development will be normal.

## HYPOTHYROIDISM: WHAT LIFE IS LIKE WITH LOW THYROID FUNCTION

Being thyroid-hormone-deficient slows down your metabolism, so you will gain weight no matter how healthy your diet. Your cholesterol levels will increase because your body cannot metabolise fats properly, and your sluggish digestion will cause constipation. You will feel tired no matter how much sleep you get and you may have less interest in sex. You will have difficulty controlling your body temperature and feel much more sensitive to heat or cold. Your hair will be dry and may thin or fall out, and your nails will become brittle. You might be prone to frequent colds and chest infections and suffer muscle aches and pains. There might be some fluid retention and puffiness. It may also become more difficult to keep up as well as you did before both physically and mentally, as thyroid deficiency can result in depression, confusion or loss of mental acuity.

These are just the most common symptoms a patient with hypothyroidism may show, but who among us has not experienced some, if not many, of them? Does this mean that we all have an under-functioning thyroid? This is a very difficult question to answer. These same symptoms can also be caused by countless other conditions – from anaemia to PMS, depression, chronic fatigue, and immunity and digestive problems.

Diagnosing the root of such problems can be confusing and frustrating for both patient and doctor. Sometimes the medical practitioner can lack the time, interest or imagination to delve into the patient's complaints. If patients say they are feeling tired or down or that they're not coping with their life, they are usually offered antidepressants as a matter of course. Or they are told to pull themselves together, eat less and exercise more. Their doctor might even explain that their fatigue, weight gain and mood swings are all part of the ageing process, and they should simply accept that they are 'slowing down'.

## THE HIDDEN DISEASE

Thyroid disease can be masked in many ways. One of the most frustrating things for patients is knowing that something is wrong and yet being dismissed by their GP. This is a familiar scenario:

a GP orders blood tests, and when the results show up as 'normal' or within the acceptable reference range, the patient is declared healthy and told to stop complaining.

The problem here is that the patient's symptoms do not correlate with the blood-test results. But who or what are we treating – the patient or the blood tests? So-called reference ranges in blood tests are basically just a series of results that have been deemed normal or healthy. When outside of these ranges, the results are considered evidence of pathology or disease, but there is another way to interpret such results. I often explain to my patients that rather than looking for simply 'normal' or 'abnormal' results, we are looking for an optimal range. We can pass an exam at 55 per cent *and* at 95 per cent. Both are a pass marks, but where would we prefer to be? We want to excel in our health.

So, I (and like-minded practitioners) interpret results somewhat differently from our peers. To my mind, patients' symptoms are paramount, and their blood tests should be understood as part of the bigger picture. Even if the blood tests come back within the normal range, I will still consider treating a patient who has physical and psychological symptoms of a disease. Of course, this can lead to a quandary when we, the consulting doctors, fall out of the range of conventional treatments with our advice and prescriptions. In other words, we do not do what our peers do and thus come in for criticism from the medical fraternity. We are always aware of this, but we are so encouraged by our patients and their good results that we decide to risk being called a 'complementary physician' or 'different type of doctor' and do it anyway.

There follow two cases where the symptoms pointed to an obvious cause, but all blood tests came back 'normal'.

# *Rhonda's story*

## OVERWEIGHT DESPITE A PERFECT DIET; THINNING HAIR

**The Hormone Doctor:** Rhonda arrived in my office short of breath after climbing one flight of stairs. Rhonda was 44 years old, had two teenage children and worked part-time in a school canteen. I noted that Rhonda looked pale, that she was slightly overweight and had very thin, dry hair. She sat down and told me that she knew something wasn't right and she felt unwell, but that all her blood tests had come back within the normal range, except for her cholesterol, which was elevated. Her GP prescribed her statins and said that was all he could do for her.

Rhonda was mainly concerned about her thinning hair. She had noticed she was losing more hair when she washed it, and every time she brushed her hair 'handfuls' came out. She told me that her mother had lost a lot of hair in her 50s, and it had never grown back; Rhonda was worried that the same was going to happen to her.

Rhonda's thyroid blood tests were 'normal': in the mid-to-low range of acceptability. But there was more to the picture than just the blood-test results – her hair loss made that clear. Her hair was thinning on the crown, and had lost its sheen and lustre. She was also easily fatigued and, although generally unfit (she was always too tired to exercise), nothing had changed in her life. Rhonda wasn't under any stress; she remarked that she was in a happy marriage, her teenage children caused her no problems and she enjoyed her work.

Her thinning hair, her fatigue, her elevated cholesterol, the pallor of her skin and her loss of stamina, coupled with her mother's history of hair loss, pointed to a sluggish if not under-functioning thyroid. I decided to treat her with a low dose of thyroxine (50 micrograms) and then monitor her response. If her thyroid was the cause of her problems, then she would see an improvement in her symptoms after one or two months of treatment. I always tell my patients that if they get some palpitations or their hands begin to shake, then the treatment I have recommended is either wrong for them or the dose is too high. If this happens, I recommend that they return for a consultation immediately so I can review their situation.

During her first two months of treatment, I also sent Rhonda to Vicki for nutritional advice regarding her weight and elevated cholesterol.

**The Nutritionist:** When I met with Rhonda and we discussed her diet, I discovered that it could not be faulted – her increased cholesterol levels could not be traced back to anything she was eating. My only advice was for her to take daily antioxidant and selenium supplements.

**The Hormone Doctor:** It was not Rhonda's diet that had affected her cholesterol; it was her subtle hypothyroidism. In fact, some researchers say that hypothyroidism can be diagnosed purely by a raised cholesterol level. When Rhonda returned to my office two months after her first appointment, she was pleased to tell me that she felt much better on her thyroid medication. She was thrilled to find that her hair had not only stopped falling out, but was even growing back. She had experienced no signs of thyroxine overmedication, such as palpitations or tremors. When I repeated her thyroid blood tests, I found that her results were now in the optimal range of healthy thyroid function and her cholesterol levels had improved. Rhonda's energy levels also improved and she started an exercise routine.

Rhonda has remained on the thyroxine medication ever since, and is now entering peri-menopause, so far with very few symptoms, a full head of hair and lots of energy.

# Andrea's story

## HAIR LOSS AND 'UTTER EXHAUSTION'

**The Hormone Doctor:** Andrea has also had a longstanding battle with her thyroid, stress levels, weight and hair. Andrea was 42, and her hypothyroidism was apparently under control – or so she was being continually told by her GP and specialist – but Andrea was not well. She found she was always pushing herself to get through the day. She was struggling to lose the weight she put on after her first child (seven years earlier), and she had lost a lot of hair – a state she hid under colourful scarves and headbands.

The first time Andrea experienced symptoms of hypothyroidism was after the birth of her first child. She had lost most of her hair in a matter of weeks and was excessively fatigued. Her doctor, who suspected postnatal depression, also decided to check her thyroid before prescribing antidepressants. He was concerned about her hair loss, which he thought was possibly caused by stress, but needed to rule out an under-functioning thyroid.

The blood test was a blessing. Andrea was not depressed. She was understandably distressed about her hair loss and felt utterly exhausted, although this was not caused by a new mother's sleepless nights as her daughter was a good sleeper from very early on. If this test had not been carried out, Andrea would have been put on antidepressants and sent on her way. She would not only have been advised against continuing to breastfeed her newborn (as antidepressants are generally not recommended for lactating women), she would also have been wrongly diagnosed.

Andrea's GP prescribed her thyroxine, which improved her energy levels and stopped her hair from falling out, but she was not given any advice regarding supplements that could support her thyroid and adrenal glands nor any nutritional recommendations. Andrea had periods of feeling 'okay'. She returned to a challenging job in PR and continued life with her demanding husband. She loved her life, but often felt she lacked the energy to enjoy what was going on around her. When stress peaked in work and family life, Andrea would experience periods of increased hair loss that would last for a few weeks at a time.

Andrea managed on the prescribed treatment but always felt that she could be better. She continually battled with her weight and lack of energy and also suffered from PMS, becoming very fatigued and irritable the week before her periods were due.

Most GPs check only TSH (thyroid-stimulating hormone) and T4 (thyroxine) levels when patients take thyroid medication. We assume that when these levels are normal then the medication is adequate, but for patients who still complain that they could or want to feel better we should also check the T3 (tri-iodothyronine, circulating thyroid hormone) levels. Andrea's T3 levels were below the normal range, an indication of Wilson's syndrome, which means that the body is unable to convert T4 into T3.

I supplemented Andrea's thyroxine medication with a small amount of T3 and it made all the difference to her energy levels and general feeling of wellbeing. (When T3 is supplemented, it is more readily absorbed and has a more rapid effect, so it needs to be monitored very closely.) I also prescribed her some progesterone cream to apply one week before her period, which reduced her irritability. She was very satisfied with this regime and remains so to this day. Of course, every six months I ask Andrea to come back so I can check her blood levels and make sure she is not overmedicated.

**The Nutritionist:** Marion referred Andrea to me to suggest ways to support her thyroid function, and to ensure that she was not eating foods or drinks that would in any way interfere with or suppress her thyroid function further.

I started by recommending that Andrea cut out all stimulants such as caffeinated drinks (tea, coffee and fizzy drinks), as these all place a burden on the adrenal glands, which then rely on the thyroid gland for support. (This is known in medical terms as the adrenal–thyroid–pituitary axis, and is a fine example of how the glands of the endocrine system work together to support the body.)

I recommended that Andrea drink rooibos (African red bush) tea, which would give an uplifting feeling without the caffeine. (Rooibos is now widely available in supermarkets and health food shops.) I also suggested an excellent South American tea called yerba maté, which is also naturally stimulating and now widely recognised for its antioxidant properties.

I felt that these substitutes were important for Andrea, as she had relied heavily on caffeine to 'keep her going' when she felt so exhausted – but in fact it was doing the exact opposite in the longer term.

In addition, I recommended that she eat plenty of sushi wrapped in nori seaweed. Nori (along with other seaweeds) is a rich source of iodine, an essential mineral for the support of the thyroid. Iodine is often lacking in modern food because most of it has been farmed out of the soil in the Western world. Iodine and zinc, which are found in shellfish, whole grains, nuts and seeds, are both vital for healthy thyroid function. I recommended that Andrea eat sushi and shellfish once a week.

Finally, I advised her which foods have a thyroid-suppressing effect – they are known as 'goitrogens', as their suppressing nature can induce a goitre in the base of the throat area, which is a sure symptom of thyroid disease. These foods, while considered healthy for most, should be restricted in anyone with an underactive thyroid. They include broccoli, cabbage, bok choy, cauliflower and Brussels sprouts – all members of the Brassicaceae family of plants. It was this last recommendation that surprised Andrea the most, as she had always eaten large amounts of all of them, believing them to be good for her. I assured her that she would be consuming the antioxidants and other important nutrients she needed from other foods in her varied diet and she agreed to comply.

Surprisingly, Andrea didn't suffer any of the usual symptoms of caffeine withdrawal – night sweats, irritability, headaches and stomach upsets – and found a new passion for rooibos tea. She felt noticeably better within a few weeks and realised what a mistake she had made by propping herself up with copious amounts of coffee and tea. Cutting out the brassica vegetables to a large extent encouraged her to look for new vegetables that she had not included in her diet previously, such as squashes, beans and root vegetables.

## WHEN THE WEIGHT DOESN'T SHIFT NO MATTER WHAT YOU DO

Two of the most common symptoms related to an underactive thyroid are unexplained weight gain or immense difficulty losing weight. This causes untold frustration for many women.

## *Roberta's story*

### YOYO-ING WEIGHT LEVELS: 'OUT OF SORTS'

**The Hormone Doctor:** Roberta was 33 years old and came to me hoping to sort out two issues. The first was a lifelong battle with her weight. The second was her blood-test results: they showed elevated thyroid-stimulating hormone (TSH) levels, which can lead to an under-functioning thyroid.

When Roberta was 14 she put on about 40 kilograms (6 stone or 88 pounds) of extra weight, but looking at her now, I found it hard to imagine. The adult I saw before me was fine-boned, with small wrists and ankles, and did not look like an obese person. But at the age of 16 she had weighed 115 kilograms (18 stone or 254 pounds).

Roberta controlled her weight – then as now – by keeping to a strict diet and regular exercise regime. Her average weight over the last 10 years had been 65 kilograms (10 stone or 143 pounds), and she was 162 centimetres (5 feet 4 inches) tall.

When Roberta was 24 she had another period of unexplained weight gain. Over just two weeks, without any change to her diet, exercise regime or stress factors, she ballooned 10 kilograms (22 pounds or 1½ stone). During this time, she felt excessively tired and 'out of sorts'. She also stated that she had experienced body aches and pain, and felt that the only thing that allowed her to function 'normally' was her exercise. She was a disciplined person, ate well and regularly, but couldn't countenance a day without exercise.

At that time, Roberta had had her thyroid checked and her borderline results meant no doctor was willing to treat her. When I saw Roberta, it had been eight years since this sudden weight gain, and she still complained of aching, swollen legs, excessive fatigue and 'brain fog'. She knew something was wrong and told me she thought it was her thyroid. Her mother and another close relative had thyroid problems and she suspected she did too.

While Roberta was telling me her story, it became obvious that she was only maintaining her energy levels and a functioning metabolism through her high levels of daily exercise. She could not stop exercising, because when she did, she would collapse in a heap. Ironically for

Roberta, taking a day off was a far more exhausting option than another day of exercise.

I suspected Roberta's thyroid *was* the culprit and sent her off for the appropriate blood tests. This time her tests were no longer borderline: they were in the abnormal range – her TSH was raised to 6.0. I prescribed Roberta a low dose of thyroxine (50 micrograms per day). Roberta was thrilled that I was willing to treat her thyroid disease, as she felt that until now her pleas had fallen on deaf ears.

The genetic component of thyroid disease is often overlooked by medical practitioners, but I believe family history should be one of the first questions asked of a patient whose symptoms align with thyroid deficiency, even if their blood-test results don't.

Roberta felt an instant improvement after taking the thyroxine. Her aches and pain receded, her 'brain fog' cleared and her energy levels improved almost immediately. With the help of Vicki's advice, her exercise regime and medication she was able to maintain her desired weight, her activities and her career.

**The Nutritionist:** Marion sent Roberta to me because of her tendency to gain weight easily. I looked at her eating plan, which was both sensible and appropriate, but I was concerned that it lacked sufficient quantities of foods containing zinc and iodine, minerals that are vital for thyroxine production.

I suggested that she take colloidal iodine drops, available from good health food shops or through qualified nutritionists. (Colloidal minerals are in a liquid form and can be absorbed through the micro-capillaries under the tongue straight into the bloodstream.) As well as the iodine, I suggested Roberta take a complex antioxidant containing high-dose zinc (50 milligrams), at night for maximum potency.

> ## Did you know . . . ?
> Mineral supplements are best absorbed when taken at night, whereas vitamin supplements are best absorbed when taken during the day.

## Alex's story

### INAPPROPRIATELY EXHAUSTED AFTER EXERCISE

**The Nutritionist:** Alex was 39, successful and energetic. She ran her own business, and had always been self-motivated. She admitted to having had problems with her weight and having been a yoyo dieter in her late teens and early 20s, but she had seen a nutritionist six years before, who had helped her sort out her diet and put her on the straight and narrow. When Alex came to see me, however, she asked me to help her figure out why, despite an eating regime that seemed to suit her energy needs and should have allowed her to lose weight, her weight had remained the same for the last 18 months. Alex was clearly quite frustrated by the situation.

Alex had always been a runner: 'I don't feel the same if I don't start the day with a run.' In addition, she usually managed to fit in at least two spin classes a week – so clearly she was getting plenty of exercise. But Alex did complain that she had recently felt inappropriately exhausted after exercise.

When I took Alex's family history, I noted that both her mother and aunt had had 'some kind of thyroid illness', although Alex was not sure what. On questioning her, I also discovered that she cried easily ('sometimes at the most ridiculous things, actually'), had itchy eyelids, and permanently cold hands and feet. All of these symptoms, when found together, can suggest an underactive thyroid.

I suggested that it would be a good idea to test Alex's thyroid function, as everything else seemed to be in balance. I referred her back to her doctor, asking him to carry out a thyroid function test.

Three weeks later, Alex returned to me in tears: 'My doctor says my thyroid is normal – so if it isn't that, what is the matter with me?' I asked her to send me a copy of the test results so I could judge for myself. As we saw in Andrea's story (page 177), the standard test for thyroid function measures TSH (thyroid-stimulating hormone) and T4 (thyroxine levels in the thyroid). The test results for Alex did indeed fall within the normal range, which showed me that she was producing sufficient thyroxine, but I still didn't know if she was actually *using* the thyroxine at a cellular level. The fact that she had been feeling more tired after exercise lately, suggested to me that something definitely wasn't right.

I sent Alex for a more detailed form of the test, which is now more readily available from most testing laboratories. Not surprisingly, Alex's levels of T3 (circulating thyroid hormone) were indeed low, which indicated that, while her thyroid was producing the necessary thyroxine, she was not able to benefit from it. In other words, she was not converting it into a bio-available form.

The conversion process of T4 to T3 requires adequate levels of selenium in the body – and selenium is notoriously deficient in most Western countries due mainly to over-farming of soils and the consumption of high junk-food diets. I recommended that Alex aim to eat selenium-rich foods every day – seafood (including fish and seaweeds – both dry and fresh), sesame seeds (mainly in the form of tahini, sesame paste), and a yeast spread such as Marmite or Vegemite. I also gave her a daily nutritional supplement of selenium to ensure that her intake would remain consistent over the next three months.

Most importantly, I asked Alex to stop drinking alcohol during that three-month period. Alcohol is a known thyroid suppressor in any quantity, particularly for someone whose thyroid function is already under par. Alex agreed to this regime and went off armed with her new information.

Four months later, Alex returned with good news – her former energy levels had returned, she had lost more than 6 kilograms and had rediscovered her waist! She had also cut back to running only four times a week rather than every day, allowing herself a sleep-in ('utter bliss!') at weekends. We retested her T3 levels and found they had returned to normal. But the real proof was in her constitution – 'I feel stronger in myself, I don't cry at the drop of a hat, and I no longer feel as if there's something wrong with me.' Another happy client!

## NUTRITIONAL ADVICE FOR BOOSTING YOUR THYROID

The most productive way to combat unexplained weight gain is to support your thyroid function. From a dietary perspective, this means eating plenty of those foods containing nutrients that support the thyroid, such as iodine, zinc and magnesium, as well as the lesser known selenium. It is also important to cut back on foods that tend to suppress thyroid function.

In order to support your thyroid, you should eat selenium-rich foods every day; these include seafood (fish and seaweeds, both dry and fresh), sesame seeds (mainly in the form of tahini – sesame seed paste), and yeast spreads such as Marmite or Vegemite.

While broccoli is a very healthy food, it belongs to the Brassicaceae family of plants, which are known to suppress thyroid function. This is not to say that you shouldn't eat brassicas, but if you suspect that you may have a marginally underactive thyroid, you should eat the following foods only occasionally rather than daily.

## Thyroid-suppressing foods

- Brussels sprouts
- broccoli, purple sprouting broccoli
- cauliflower
- cabbage (all types, including Chinese leaf)
- turnips
- swedes

Research has shown that in some people the protein found in wheat, called gliadin, can produce a similar effect to the antibodies that attack the thyroid gland in autoimmune conditions. While one condition has nothing to do with the other, the symptoms are often the same – fatigue, loss of enthusiasm, mild to moderate depression, unexplained weight gain and hair loss. In cases where these symptoms are present but thyroid tests all prove to be normal, I always recommend that my clients have a gliadin sensitivity test. It is not so difficult nowadays to cut down on, or cut out of your diet altogether, refined-wheat products, as there are many alternatives to this overused grain product.

Most importantly, though, if you are suffering from an under-active thyroid, you should be very wary of alcohol. Alcohol in any quantity is a known thyroid suppressor, and is particularly bad for those whose thyroid function is already suboptimal.

Some foods and nutrients are known to boost thyroid activity, so include plenty of the following thyroid megafoods and nutrients in your diet.

## Thyroid megafoods

- calf and chicken livers (vitamin A)
- lean meats, dairy produce (B12)
- seafood, shellfish, poultry, lean meat, whole grains (zinc)
- nuts and seeds (selenium, zinc and B vitamins)
- kiwifruit, sweet potatoes, green leafy vegetables (vitamin C)

## Thyroid meganutrients

A daily dose of high-quality colloidal minerals including zinc and selenium, taken with a B-complex vitamin and a broad-spectrum antioxidant (to cover vitamins A, C and E), will ensure you receive all of these vital nutrients. There are a number of specific thyroid-supportive nutritional supplements on the market.

| Nutrient | Function |
|---|---|
| Vitamin A (not alpha- and beta-carotene alone, as these are not converted effectively in cases of underactive thyroid) | Essential for the production of TSH and to convert T4 into T3 |
| Vitamin B5 (pantothenic acid) | Required for the adrenal glands |
| Vitamin B6 | To convert iodine into thyroid hormones |
| Vitamin B12 (best absorbed in blue-green algae or chlorella formulations) | Required for protein digestion |
| Vitamin C | Required for thyroid and adrenal support |
| Vitamins D and E | These vitamins are depleted from other organs in the body in people with overactive thyroid problems |
| Magnesium | Needed to convert T4 into T3, as well as for supporting the adrenal glands |
| Selenium | Imperative for the conversion of T4 into T3; selenium deficiency can produce a false 'normal' level of hormones in a thyroid-function blood test |
| Zinc | Needed to convert T4 into T3 |

## WHEN THE BURPS GET BEYOND A JOKE

Bloating, wind, burping, heartburn, constipation and abdominal discomfort are all common complaints of women with hormone imbalances. The ramifications of this are wider reaching than you might realise. After food is broken down in your mouth and passed to your stomach, your stomach acid breaks down proteins *before* they reach your small intestine. If there is insufficient stomach acid to break down the proteins, then the minerals contained in those protein foods cannot be absorbed properly in the small intestine. It's all very well to ensure you are eating foods rich in calcium, magnesium and manganese for bone and ligament health, but it's no use if you can't extract and absorb those minerals after you've eaten them.

But how does this relate to thyroid function? First, an underactive thyroid has a direct effect on the production of hydrochloric acid in the stomach, as well as digestive enzymes in the pancreas and elsewhere in the digestive tract, all of which are linked hormonally. Secondly, if you have been suffering from chronic stress (severe allergies or intolerances, chronic pain or long-term medication) or a massive shock (loss of a loved one, divorce, being made redundant, and so on), your adrenal glands – your stress-regulators – will be working overtime. When they are under pressure, the adrenal glands suppress the production of stomach acid in the stomach and – voilà! – indigestion. The adrenal glands and the thyroid work in tandem – if one is overworked, the other will help to take the strain. This is a fantastic example of how intricately interwoven the endocrine glands are.

In dealing with indigestion, I recommend that my clients look at how and when they eat their meals: eating on the run is absolutely forbidden – I ask them to take at least 20 minutes over each meal. I also suggest that they regularly use stimulating herbs and spices, such as turmeric, cumin, paprika, cayenne pepper and finely ground black pepper, in their recipes. These all stimulate the digestion to work more efficiently. It's also a good idea to start every day with a large mug of hot water, grated ginger and the juice of half a lemon, as this will help stimulate stomach acid. It's also great for flushing out the liver.

## Digestion megafoods

| Food | Good for ... |
|---|---|
| Cooked garlic and onions | Support the production of bile salts by the liver |
| Apples, papaya, pears, pineapples, mangoes, blueberries | Contain digestive enzymes that support the production of pancreatic enzymes |
| Avocados | Rich in vitamin E, which reduces inflammation in the small and large intestines |
| Fennel and dandelion flowers | Anti-spasmodic effect |
| Celery | Enhances digestion in the stomach |
| Asparagus | Diuretic |

*Did you know . . . ?*

From our mid-30s onwards, the natural production of stomach acid starts to diminish. By the time we are in our late 40s or early 50s, most women (and men) produce less than half the stomach acid they did in their 20s. It's little wonder we end up with indigestion!

## ALL BLOCKED UP

It seems that not only do French women not get fat, they also don't get blocked up. People seem fascinated by the topic and yet so few have adopted a Frenchwoman's strategies. First, French women generally take greater care with their health and their appearance than most. But more importantly, they all know how vital digestive health is for maintaining a flat abdomen, banishing bloating and preventing constipation. You can keep up your punishing sit-up regime all you like, but it won't give you the washboard stomach of your 20s if your digestion isn't working properly.

The thyroid directly affects our large intestine (colon) by stimulating peristalsis (the strong muscular actions that move faecal matter through to the bowel), and as such is responsible for whether we become constipated. It is not uncommon for peri-menopausal and menopausal women to develop constipation, from which they might never have suffered before. This is a result of lowered levels of oestrogen and sluggish thyroid function. I'm certain many women on conventional HRT are still suffering constipation, since replacing lost oestrogen is only half the equation – the second actor in the play is the thyroid, and this is often overlooked.

In France a pharmacist will supply probiotics to accompany any prescribed course of antibiotics. Antibiotics kill off pathogens (invading bacteria), but they also kill off the beneficial bacteria that live in the large intestine. These good bacteria help us to digest residual food and support a hearty immune system. It is often said that 'death begins in the colon', but ensuring that the large intestine has plenty of beneficial bacteria is one of the best preventative measures you can take against constipation and more serious long-term illnesses such as diverticulitis, polyps and even colon cancer.

If you suffer from constipation, I recommend soaking oats overnight in a mixture of half apple juice and half water to create a delicious morning muesli (this was the original recipe for Bircher muesli, which came from the Bircher-Brenner naturopathic clinic in Germany). Stir in 1 tablespoon of ground linseed just before you eat the muesli. Linseed, in addition to being a good source of phyto-hormones, acts like a broom for the intestines. (It is not recommended, however, for those who have any form of intestinal inflammation, for example Crohn's disease or ulcerative colitis.)

To combat constipation, you should be eating plenty of green vegetables (up to 1 kilogram, or 2 pounds, daily). Especially good are zucchini (courgettes), asparagus, French beans, runner beans, cucumber and snow peas (mange tout). Steam these vegetables for no more than three minutes – just enough time to make them more easily digestible while not stripping away any of their nutritional content. They will provide plenty of fibre in a form that will not cause constipation but instead rehydrate the large intestine and bowel. This is a more effective way to treat constipation than eating copious salads and raw vegetables, which your body may not be able to break down properly, thus causing further discomfort and bloating. Once your bowel is functioning well, you can reintroduce salads and raw vegetables to your diet.

---

### Did you know . . . ?

The amount of sugar in so-called probiotic yoghurts or yoghurt drinks negates any benefit the probiotics can give you. Don't get sucked into this marketing ploy!

---

## MANAGING WEIGHT GAIN IN MENOPAUSE

By far the loudest complaints menopausal women make are about weight gain – 'I never used to have this bulge', or 'I may have put on weight over the years, but this is out of control' or even 'I don't recognise myself any more; I'm 49 and I look like I did when I was six months pregnant!'. Often the first question women ask regarding a particular treatment is 'But will this help me to lose weight?'.

With the dramatic hormonal changes that take place during

peri-menopause and menopause, our metabolic rate changes and weight gain is, sadly, almost inevitable. While certain diets *may* have worked for you in the past, you may now find that your body is no longer responsive. Why is this?

Your thyroid, which regulates your metabolism, is sensitive to changes in calorie intake and to changes in the ratio of proteins, carbohydrates and fats. The yoyo approach of dieting and bingeing over a number of years, however, causes the thyroid to become less sensitive to such changes, making it difficult to lose any weight at all. For some, it seems as though eating *anything* leads to weight gain. This is intensely frustrating for many women and one of the hardest menopausal symptoms to deal with.

So what is a healthy approach to dieting in menopause?

## BAN THE CALORIE COUNT

Calories were devised as a calculation of how much energy each food could yield (in measurable units). Accordingly, those foods that are high in protein and fats, such as red meat and dairy produce, are inevitably high in calories, as they take longer to digest than grains or vegetables and produce a prolonged source of energy. Such foods are also considered to be 'fattening' and are recognised contributors to heart disease. An avocado, which is often avoided by dieters for its calorie-richness, provides a good level of energy, as it contains more protein than almost any other fruit (proteins take longer to break down and absorb than carbohydrates). Both options are considered to be 'high in calories', but this doesn't mean that both are bad for you.

As a nutritionist, I disregard calorie counting and look instead for the energy and nutritional values in each food. To this end, I suggest that you eat a serving of lean red meat once or twice a week for its high levels of iron and other important minerals, and happily recommend eating four or five avocados a week, as they are an excellent vegetarian source of protein and rich in essential fatty acids and vitamin E, which keeps your skin supple and youthful.

Far too much time is spent agonising over the calorie count of food products, and people too often favour low-fat choices because they keep the overall count down. Remember, though, that when you choose a 'low-fat' or 'no-fat' product (particularly those that would normally have contained a certain amount of fat, such as yoghurt) that product will have had other ingredients added to make up the total weight of the original *before* the fat was removed. The most likely ingredients are sugar and salt, and the irony is that all added sugars are converted into fat. You might have chosen a product with its original fat removed, but that very product will contain enough sugar to be converted into fat in its end stage of digestion and absorption.

While saturated fat (found in meats and dairy produce) is potentially damaging to the cardiovascular system when eaten in excess, the essential fats found in fish, nuts, seeds (and their oils) work in precisely the opposite way. They reduce inflammation, protect against dehydration of the skin and internal organs, and are essential for nerve transmission – helping to protect memory and cognitive function. Most importantly, these essential fatty acids help us *break down* excess stored fat and *lose* it! This is the very reason why low-fat, no-fat diets do not work – because *some* of the right fats are important in our diets, especially when we reach menopause and our oestrogen levels are dropping.

## CHEMICALS – THE HORMONE DISRUPTORS

One of the most important areas of nutrition to address at this stage in life is the *quality* of your food. There are three main times in life when eating good-quality food is more than just important, it is essential: during childhood, when the body and brain are developing; during pregnancy, when you are developing a whole new life in your body; and during the menopausal years, when the process of biological repair is slowing down and your immune system needs to be in peak health to prevent the onset of disease.

How often do you eat something only to notice that your hands or ankles have become puffy within half an hour of finishing your meal? Or that your skin has started itching for no apparent reason? Or that it leads to a headache when this has never been a problem for you before? The explanation may partly involve your changing hormone levels, but it could also relate to a chemical sensitivity.

Chemicals are commonplace in most pre-prepared, pre-cooked and pre-packed meals and snacks. While these days we have ready access to options that use only natural preservatives, sweeteners and colourings, these are more expensive. Cheaper mainstream food choices still use an array of chemicals that are foreign to our bodies. During and after menopause, women tend to be far more sensitive to the chemical onslaught they might have tolerated in their younger years. Our liver, the main organ of detoxification in the body, can no longer break down these chemicals as efficiently. The most common reactions to food chemicals are fluid retention and weight gain. When you jump on the scales in the morning, despairing at that extra weight that appeared overnight, you should not be asking yourself whether you ate too much, but instead what was *in* your food.

Perhaps the pre-prepared meal you heated up in the oven had too much salt in it. Or it might have included a raft of chemicals not even listed on the packaging because their percentage in the overall dish was relatively negligible but still enough to ruin your day.

My rule of thumb is simple – if you eat food 'as nature intended', your body will know what to do with it, and there will be no residues of additives, sweeteners or other chemicals to disrupt your hormones or end up being stored in fatty tissue. Chemicals in foods overload the liver's detoxification processes, interfering with its ability to break down oestrogen.

# Davina's story

## WEIGHT GAIN: 'I NEVER DREAMED I'D LOOK LIKE THIS!'

**The Nutritionist:** Davina was a strong, vibrant, good-looking woman in her late-50s. She came to see me because she had put on more than 20 kilograms (44 pounds or 3 stone) over the last five or six years. 'I knew my body might change as I got older, but I never dreamed I'd end up looking like this!' she lamented. Though she had never been petite, she was distressed that menopause had left her with a thickened waistline, saggy bottom and flabby arms.

Davina correctly recognised that some of this had to do with hormonal changes, but during our consultation it emerged that her weight gain was in large part a result of her diet. 'I used to eat so well – all through my teens, my 20s, my pregnancies and well into my 40s. But recently I've just let go. I feel as though I have cooked enough dinners for a lifetime, and the ease of a dinner I can just unwrap and put into the oven is too tempting to resist.' Understandably, now that only Davina and her husband were left in the family home, her incentive to cook had waned. Changes in Davina's snacking habits had occurred too; her favourites now consisted of anything 'doughy, sugary and sweet'.

I pointed out a simple fact not known to many women – sugar is addictive. Actually, it's a cumulative addiction. The bacteria in the large intestine that feed on sugars can proliferate and subsequently become 'hungrier' for more sugars. Many people find themselves saying that they don't know what to do, that they seem to have no control over their eating habits. It is not a matter of weak will on their part – the pathogenic bacteria are placing increasing demands on their diet. And things get harder for women during and after menopause because their body's digestive function slows down and declines in efficiency, meaning these bacteria can proliferate further.

I helped Davina to work out an eating program that resembled how she ate during her 20s and 30s. I reminded her that most of her food intake at that stage of her life would have been in a more natural form, comprising fish, poultry, lean red meat and fresh vegetables. Pre-packed dinner meals were not so readily available then, nor were the many cakes, snacks and fast food she had become so dependent on to 'relieve her fatigue'. These foods, packed with unhealthy simple carbohydrates, were in fact at the very core of perpetuating her fatigue, so I persuaded her to include more complex carbohydrates in her diet, in the form of brown rice, barley and porridge oats.

Davina came back to see me some months later. Not surprisingly, she got on well with her old program – her body had responded within the first two weeks, shedding 2.7 kilograms (6 pounds). Feeling inspired, she took up horse riding (something she hadn't done in 10 years), and found that the weight continued to drop off at the same rate for the next six weeks before evening out. 'I couldn't believe it could have been that simple – why didn't I think of that?'

Davina's story illustrates the essence of my advice to most of my menopausal clients: go back to how you ate in your teens and 20s and your body will follow suit – your spare tyre will disappear, your batwings will shrink (although you'll need some toning from swimming, Pilates or yoga), and your bottom will lose most of its dimples.

## KEEP IT LEAN, KEEP IT CLEAN, KEEP IT GREEN

Research is now showing that staying lean keeps us younger longer, and that weight management isn't about reducing the number of calories you consume, it's about the quality of the nutrients in the food you're eating. Choosing lean forms of animal protein, such as fish, game birds, turkey, eggs and lean red meat, is important, as protein should form between 35 and 40 per cent of your daily intake. But not all protein need be from animal sources; you should include sprouted beans, seeds and grains, as well as nuts and seeds, pulses and soy-based foods – in that order.

Skipping breakfast altogether is a big no-no. You will never lose weight the way you want to by skipping breakfast. Grains are important in your diet for adequate amounts of energy-producing B vitamins, but they don't suit everyone, and it appears that women can find grains more difficult to digest as they get older. This is one of the reasons I don't advocate eating muesli (apart from Bircher muesli) or porridge for breakfast – I know that they make many women feel bloated and hungry for the rest of the day. It's far better to start the day with lean protein, such as eggs or fish, with a small portion of a whole-grain or pumpernickel bread, or a fruit smoothie made with a combination of ground nuts, seeds and a nut milk (almond milk, for example) or soy milk. Protein in the morning raises your metabolic rate for several hours after the meal, and gives you lasting energy.

I generally recommend that no more than 15 per cent of your daily food intake be grain-based – be it cereals, breads, rice or couscous. If you're serious about managing your weight and fat distribution, you should omit grains from your evening meal – any starch eaten at night that exceeds your energy needs will be converted into fat.

Eating more vegetables and less fruit is another key recommendation: fruit is good for you, of course, but too much fruit simply overloads your body with excess sugars (albeit natural sugars), and upsets your sugar regulation. So many people take their 'five-a-day' fruit and vegetable recommendation to mean three or four portions of fruit and one or two of vegetables. I persuade my patients to have one portion of fruit and four portions of vegetables and salad leaves.

In fact, I work with them until they are eating nearer to 10–12 portions a day, and only two of those portions are fruit.

Fruit and vegetables should occupy at least 40–50 per cent of your total daily food intake. Variety is the key here: aim for a rainbow of colours on your plate or in your bowl at every meal. Be bold and seek out varieties you haven't eaten in years, rather than following culinary fashions. Rocket and watercress are indeed good for you, but so too are kale, Savoy cabbage, fennel and celery. You will see throughout this book that I recommend certain foods for multiple conditions because of their specific hormone-balancing or hormone-supportive nutrients. This doesn't mean, however, that these should be the only foods you choose – be adventurous and your body (and metabolism) will respond to the challenge. Take a look at these five key guidelines for controlling your weight.

---

**Five guidelines for weight management**

1. Eat food as nature intended – avoid low-fat or no-fat options
2. Keep it lean, keep it clean, keep it green
3. Eat adequate quantities of animal and vegetable proteins at every meal
4. Avoid starches (grains) with your evening meal
5. Cut out all sugars, additives, preservatives and other chemicals

---

Food diaries are a nightmare for some, but they are a good way to reveal patterns in your eating and drinking. Once you have identified your 'addictions', your 'repetitions' and your 'fake foods and drinks', it's then simpler to go back to the 'as nature intended' alternatives. I maintain that keeping and examining a food diary is the first step towards change – keep one for two weeks, and then take a stark look at what you are consuming. You might not be so surprised that your body has changed once you see what you are putting into it.

## BLOATING

Bloating occurs when the pathogenic bacteria start to outstrip the beneficial ones. It's literally a battle of good against evil and, indeed, at times it can feel as if there's a war going on down there. What is actually occurring is a process of fermentation, which causes the bloating by leading to a build-up of wind in the colon behind compacted faecal matter.

Consumption of refined carbohydrates (white bread, white rice and all commercial cakes, biscuits, bagels, doughnuts and so on) and even a 'healthy' intake of fresh fruit and fruit juices, can be culprits in this fermentation process, simply because the sugars produced by their digestion feed the bacteria in the gut and are all the more readily absorbed when there is a lack of fibre to slow absorption down. The bacteria in the large intestine then cause bloating and wind. The combination of refined carbohydrates and fruit sugars together (think white toast and jam) is disastrous.

Coffee is also a major trigger for bloating. Although many women swear by its stimulating action on the large intestine, caffeine in fact has been found to cause the villi in the intestinal tract to atrophy. The villi are the millions of finger-like projections that absorb nutrients from your food and pass them into the bloodstream. Drinking coffee before or after a meal will suppress your total digestive function and negate the benefits of many of the nutrients in your meal. What a waste! On the other hand, a small black coffee drunk on an empty stomach before exercise has been shown to increase the metabolism and fat burning for a longer period than if no coffee is drunk at all – so in the case of coffee, it's a question of what you drink and when.

> *Did you know . . . ?*
> If you become bloated immediately after eating or drinking, it is a symptom of low stomach acid. Taking digestive enzymes with added hydrochloric acid helps combat this.

## INFERTILITY

It's unfortunate that infertility has become so common a problem, but I am wary of the new medical industry that has been built around it. I have seen many patients diagnosed with infertility who have gone through IVF treatments, some successful, others not. I've also seen patients who have become pregnant after treatment of their thyroid condition or after a course of progesterone treatment. Some of the fertility patients who have come to me have failed to conceive, others have had multiple miscarriages, but all too many of them have been offered IVF treatment before the cause of their infertility has been properly investigated.

Fear of not being able to conceive is instilled in so many couples. As the trend for later-life pregnancies continues, women are constantly bombarded with statements like, 'You're getting too old', 'You won't have any eggs left', 'You'll never be able to get pregnant naturally', 'This may be your last chance', and so on. All this may be true, but sometimes the easiest solutions are not considered first. My fertility patients usually want to have a child naturally or have gone through failed IVF attempts and are hoping that they might still find a way to conceive.

I recently received a lovely email from one of my patients with a baby picture attached, thanking me for treating her thyroid and informing me that she was pregnant again. This was such a delightful surprise and what really makes my work so rewarding. So this is Joelle's story.

# Joelle's story

## TWO YEARS TRYING FOR A BABY

**The Hormone Doctor:** Joelle was in her early 30s. She and her husband had been trying to conceive for two years. Joelle's life was not particularly stressful, but she was becoming concerned that there might be a fertility problem. She had seen her GP, who referred her to an IVF clinic. She and her husband wanted to avoid IVF, so Joelle came to see me about her 'infertility problem'.

Joelle told me that her periods were always fairly regular, and that she didn't have bad premenstrual symptoms. She did, however, reveal that at times she suffered from excessive fatigue and an inability to focus or concentrate. She recalled that she had always felt tired, but now it seemed to be getting worse. Besides fatigue and 'brain fog', she also had some other symptoms, such as always feeling cold and having dry skin. Her GP had tested her thyroid function and iron levels (to exclude anaemia) and told Joelle that everything was normal.

I repeated her blood tests. My thyroid testing is more extensive than a regular GP's. It is common for T3 levels to be low (see Andrea's story on page 177), even though TSH (thyroid-stimulating hormone) and thyroxine (T4) levels look to be normal. Joelle's tests showed she wasn't anaemic and that although her thyroid-function tests were in the 'normal' range, they were at the lower end. I consider this a sub-clinical case of under-functioning thyroid.

I decided to supplement Joelle with a very low dose of a thyroid extract containing a combination of T4 and T3. If she responded well to the thyroid extract and her fatigue and other symptoms improved, then I could be sure we were on the right track. It is known that thyroid disease may contribute to infertility, but we tend only to treat the thyroid when we have clinical evidence that it is not functioning properly. Some doctors may forget the importance of looking for the physical signs and symptoms that we learned about during our university years. Today we are frightened; we practise defensive medicine to the detriment of patients instead of using our judgement and common sense. We rarely acknowledge that the patient is unwell unless we can prove it through conventional means.

Joelle came back to me a few months later feeling more energetic, and her next blood test showed that her thyroid function had improved significantly. I then left her in the care of her GP. Later on, I was thrilled to receive an email from her telling me about her baby who was now eight months old, and that she now found herself with an unexpected second pregnancy. Joelle wrote that she was convinced that her thyroid had been the cause of her 'infertility', and she was glad not to have gone down the IVF route.

Of course, I cannot prove that treating Joelle's thyroid function led to her successful pregnancies, but hers is not an isolated case. We know that the thyroid can have an effect on fertility, and we must consider this and other treatable causes before advising a patient to go for IVF. IVF is a marvellous opportunity for all those women who need it, but it is an expensive and highly stressful procedure that really should be a last resort.

## Audrey's story

### FIVE YEARS TRYING FOR A BABY

**The Hormone Doctor:** Audrey was referred to me by a women's clinic specialising in natural fertility. The clinic was made up of midwives, homeopaths, nutritionists, TCM (traditional Chinese medicine) practitioners, counsellors, yoga teachers, herbalists and a radiologist. You could call it a true 'holistic' centre dedicated to pre-conception care and fertility problems.

Audrey was in her late 30s and was desperate to have a child; she told me she had tried everything except IVF. Over the last five years during which she had been trying to conceive, Audrey had suffered six miscarriages, all of them around the sixth week of pregnancy (except for one pregnancy that had to be terminated for medical reasons). It was obvious that Audrey had no problem conceiving; her problem was maintaining a pregnancy.

Audrey had been well looked after at the fertility clinic, and they recognised that progesterone, or a lack of it, may have been the cause of her problem (read more about progesterone in Chapter 4). Progesterone is the 'pro-gestation' hormone, and no pregnancy is viable without it. The high levels of progesterone early in pregnancy may cause nausea in the first three months. Progesterone can only be prescribed by a medical doctor, and this was the reason the clinic had referred her to me.

Audrey's history was typical for progesterone deficiency and I did not hesitate to prescribe it to her. But first of all I sent her to have an ovarian ultrasound, which confirmed that she was ovulating. From this information, we could confirm that Audrey was indeed having intercourse at the right time in her cycle. I prescribed progesterone for Audrey to take from mid-cycle (day 14) until the start of her period.

Audrey conceived again after about four months of treatment. As soon as her pregnancy was confirmed, her gynaecologist took over her care. Audrey kept up her progesterone for the first trimester, until her gynaecologist was certain that the pregnancy was healthy and viable. All went well and Audrey gave birth to a healthy little girl, albeit four weeks prematurely.

## NUTRITIONAL ADVICE FOR THE BEST CHANCE OF CONCEPTION

Infertility is a growing problem in the Western world, in part because women and men now attempt to start a family much later, but also for myriad other reasons. We do know that imbalanced hormones, stress, and other environmental and behavioural factors can interfere with the ability of men and women to conceive. From a nutritionist's perspective, I encourage those with infertility problems to look carefully at pre-conceptual care – the foods they eat, the exercise they take and the lifestyle they lead. 'Preparing' for a baby should be a conscious effort for both parties involved – after all, each is making as much of a biological contribution as the other.

Isn't life a miracle? One egg and one sperm, and you've created an entire human being. But it would be wrong to think that this is *all* it takes to create a healthy baby – it also takes a multitude of proteins (amino acids), minerals, vitamins, essential fatty acids and hormones, coupled with rest, sleep and the right amount of daily exercise.

So let's look at the best ways to aid fertility through nutrition. The most important nutrient is protein, from which the very building blocks of life are derived. All animal proteins are considered 'complete proteins'; that is, they contain the eight amino acids we cannot manufacture in the body and must consume as part of our daily diet. They include poultry and eggs, lean red meat, fish, shellfish, and dairy produce from cows, sheep, goats and buffaloes.

Then there are the vegetable proteins – seeds and nuts, pulses and grains. These small seeds, which contain abundant potential for growth and life in plants, are vital for the growth of a child. A combination of animal and vegetable proteins is the ultimate recipe for life, but vegetarians can ensure the growth of a healthy baby with the right mix of nuts, seeds, pulses and soy-based foods. Interestingly the soy bean is the only vegetable-based protein that contains all eight essential amino acids, so soy products (soy milk, tofu, miso and tempeh) should form an integral part of any vegetarian's pre-conceptual plan. Sprouted beans, nuts and seeds contain higher levels of amino acids, as they are thought of as 'living foods'; that is, they have sprouted a shoot and a root, and are actively growing. They are also much tastier than their dried versions – eat them daily in salads or add them to stir-fries for variety.

Essential fats are the next most vital nutrient for ensuring your baby's development, so a low-fat or no-fat pre-conception diet is not only unhelpful, but may even be irresponsible. Every cell in our body is enclosed by a membrane made up of omega-3, -6 and -9 fatty acids. These are found in all nuts and seeds, seafood, as well as some dairy products. Goat's milk, for example, has an almost identical balance of omega-3 and -6 essential fats to human breast milk, with a relatively low saturated-fat content. This means it is well absorbed by the mother, and able to be utilised fully by the developing baby. (This, incidentally, is the best form of dairy for pregnant or breast-feeding mothers for the same reason, and it also helps to prevent dry-skin conditions in the baby, such as eczema and cradle-cap.)

A word of warning for those who cannot resist a full fried breakfast (or any other fried food): know that these vital essential fats are damaged when food is cooked at high temperatures. Frying or deep-frying not only strips away the nutritional content of essential fats, but actually makes them potentially harmful by turning them into damaging trans fats. My advice is simple – avoid all fried foods during pre-conceptual care, pregnancy and breastfeeding for the optimal health of you and your baby.

As a group, B vitamins are vital for all growth, but the most important of them is folic acid. This is critical for the development of the spinal cord and the entire neurological system. Without sufficient supplies of folic acid from the mother's stores, the risk of neurological disorders such as spina bifida is greatly increased. The medical recommendation for pregnant women is to take 400 IUs of folic acid daily, but nutritionists will often recommend double that amount, which is still within safe limits and ensures that there is enough for the mother's digestive tract to absorb. Foods that are richest in folic acid are the dark-green leafy vegetables, including curly kale, spinach, asparagus, Savoy cabbage, spring greens, broccoli and peas. It is also found in abundance in yeast extracts such as Marmite or Vegemite.

Zinc deficiency can be a nutritional cause of infertility. Women who have been on the contraceptive pill for a significant amount of time can have depleted zinc levels. Zinc is found in whole grains such as barley, brown rice, millet and oats, all shellfish and fish, red meat, poultry and eggs, cheese, milk and natural live yoghurt. For women who have been on the pill for longer than three years, however, I usually recommend 30 milligrams of zinc daily for three to six months.

Iron-deficiency anaemia can affect your ability to conceive. If you are having trouble conceiving and have been vegetarian for a number of years or have suffered from anaemia in the past, you should have a blood test to determine whether your iron levels may be a contributing factor. Iron-rich foods to include in your diet on a daily basis include apricots, prunes, raisins, dark-green leafy vegetables such as curly kale, watercress, parsley, and coriander, Savoy cabbage, rocket and Brussels sprouts. A colloidal iron supplement is preferable to ferrous sulphate (the usual recommendation of most doctors), which is not well absorbed and can cause constipation.

## JUMPING THE GUN WITH FERTILITY TREATMENT

I have frequently observed that women are offered fertility treatment long before all other options have been exhausted. This is illustrated by the following story.

## *Xenia's story*

### INABILITY TO CONCEIVE AND A FALSE DIAGNOSIS

**The Hormone Doctor:** Xenia was 33 years old when she started planning for a family. She was a busy woman who travelled widely and often for her marketing consultancy job. Her two main ambitions were to succeed in her job and to be a mother. She had been pregnant once in her early 20s but had had a termination.

After trying for two years to conceive, Xenia decided to consult a fertility specialist, who immediately recommended that she have fertility treatment – she was now 36 years old and 'time was running out'. Xenia was reluctant to try this option but was given the impression that it was her only chance. She underwent three cycles of IVF treatment, none of which was successful. At that time, she had to move overseas to Japan for her husband's job, giving up her own job to concentrate on her health and having a baby. This also gave her the time and freedom to undertake a second university degree.

While in Japan, Xenia once again consulted a fertility specialist. This specialist was somewhat discouraging, and after doing a series of blood tests diagnosed her with premature ovarian failure. This was devastating news for Xenia, who was now 38. She was put on Premarin and Provera as HRT and was advised that pregnancy was no longer an option – premature ovarian failure meant that she could not produce any eggs. This would preclude her from getting pregnant naturally, and from fertility treatment.

Xenia worked on coming to terms with the fact that not only would she never have a child, but that she was now post-menopausal. At the age of 41, Xenia moved to the UK and went to see a gynaecologist who asked that she have a pelvic ultrasound as part of her routine check-up. During the examination, the ultrasound technician com-mented that there was a follicle and that she was ovulating. Xenia was incredulous at this statement, having been told that she would never ovulate again. She began to doubt the medical treatment she'd received, and went online to do her own research. That's when she found me. She came to see me with an armful of ultrasound pictures and a huge question – 'How can this be possible?'

I explained to her that the medical fraternity will often go to the end of the spectrum before exploring the other possible causes. I was taught at medical school that when you try to diagnose a complex issue you should always consider the common causes first. Today, we no longer do this – we go head-on, moving far too quickly, recommending the shortest route to successful treatment.

Xenia was confused. She had already resigned herself to being post-menopausal and now the door had opened to other possibilities. When I first saw her, I took her off all the HRT so that I could see her situation unmasked by other treatments. When Xenia returned four weeks later, she told me she'd had her period shortly after coming off the hormone replacement. Subsequent blood tests confirmed that her levels of FSH (follicle-stimulating hormone) were in the normal range, implying that she was not post-menopausal in any way. Since that time, she has seen her gynaecologist, who confirmed the test results but told her that although she has follicles, the likelihood of her falling pregnant naturally is still slim.

Now Xenia is feeling hopeful but also has an acute sense of lost time due to her false diagnosis. Her desire to have a child is as strong as ever, though, and she is now willing to look at all possible ways to achieve her goal. She is presently on progesterone treatment and is discussing other avenues with her fertility doctor.

# 7

# all about andropause

## THE MALE VERSION OF MENOPAUSE

As the joke goes, the older you get, the smaller the balls become. You start off with football, then tennis and end up with golf.

We've all heard the jokes and stories about men and mid-life crises – plenty of them involving husbands who have traded in their cars and wives for 'newer models', who have quit their jobs to tour the country on their new Harley-Davidson motorcycles, or who have developed strange new hobbies and exchanged the family sedan for a two-seater red sports car. Sadly, such crises are no real laughing matter. A mid-life crisis can actually mean a period of intense upheaval and confusion in a man's life. Men can find themselves with an uncontrollable temper or with feelings of discontent or depression. This state of affairs can also disrupt his work and career, and have a negative impact on his ability to be a good husband, father and friend.

Although I run a women's health practice, I also treat many men and it is not unusual for women to ask me to treat their partners. Some women say that their partners have even worse hot flushes than they do or are suffering from terrible mood swings or excessive fatigue. They complain of their husbands having low libido or sexual and erectile dysfunction, or just being plain miserable to live with.

Hormones are just as important for men as they are for women, and in fact both sexes produce exactly the same hormones, just in different concentrations. Just as it is with women, hormone levels in men decline as they get older. 'Andropause', the male equivalent to menopause, usually occurs from a man's early 40s onwards.

One of the first signs is a loss of *joie de vivre*. Men may lose their stamina or motivation. They may begin to question their lives, their relationships and their work. It is not uncommon for this to happen around the same time as their wives are experiencing menopausal or peri-menopausal symptoms. During this time, both men and women may gain weight around their middle.

Male hormone issues can affect many areas of men's health. In addition to depressive moods, low libido, erectile dysfunction, hot flushes, insomnia and muscle wasting, sometimes chronic illnesses come along for the ride too – hypertension, diabetes and high cholesterol levels.

Some men lose their confidence during andropause, and it is not unusual to hear stories of men straying at this point in their life. It's not wise to speculate about the causes of infidelity, nor is it wise to deal in generalisations, since every case is unique, but as a doctor I have often observed that when hormones are on the decline, men are more likely to look for admiration outside their existing relationships, thinking this will revive their waning libido. (Why men don't delete incriminating text and email messages while they're about it, though, beggars belief.)

Women are affected differently. When their hormone levels drop, they feel less secure about their looks and often retreat, psychologically and physically, from their partners.

So how do these hormones we've already heard so much about affect men?

## TESTOSTERONE IMBALANCE

Testosterone is one of the most important hormones for men and, as we have seen, is also required by women. It fulfils many crucial functions in the body (see Chapter 5), but is most important for the healthy development of the heart. We know the heart is greatly affected by testosterone because there are more testosterone receptor sites in heart muscle than in any other muscle in the body.

Testosterone can also prevent and even reverse osteoporosis. Although osteoporosis occurs less frequently in men than it does in women, it is by no means uncommon in men. If men do develop osteoporosis, the results are often far more severe and disabling than in women. Studies have shown that men have a much higher mortality rate than women after suffering hip fractures – a common osteoporotic ailment. Muscle wasting is another consequence of low testosterone levels. Testosterone replacement can help muscle regeneration and restore strength and energy.

Lower testosterone levels in men can lead to depression and a general lack of energy. Research is still in its early stages, but testosterone may also play a major role in the prevention of Alzheimer's disease.

## DHEA: THE GREAT MOTIVATOR

The hormone DHEA (dihydroepiandrosterone) is produced mainly in the adrenal glands, with a small amount produced in the testicles. I call DHEA the *'joie de vivre* hormone', as it gives both men and women a sense of vitality, energy, drive and motivation. We have it in abundance in our youth. Production peaks in our 20s and steadily declines from then on, leaving us with very low levels by the age of 60. It is often described in popular health books as an 'anti-ageing' or 'mother' hormone, as the body can convert it into oestradiol, progesterone or testosterone as required. People who have high levels of DHEA seem to enjoy a longer lifespan and tend to age better.

## OESTROGEN AND PROGESTERONE IMBALANCE

Oestrogen and progesterone also play significant roles, although most men are not even aware that they produce these hormones and are not always happy to hear that they do. Both men and women are surprised to learn that in a couple aged 60-plus, the man may have more oestrogen in his body than the woman.

In men, progesterone acts as an aromatase-inhibitor. Aromatase is an enzyme that converts testosterone into oestradiol, and it's not a good thing for men to have too much oestradiol in their system. We know that oestradiol can cause an enlarged prostate, or prostate cancer, and high levels of oestradiol are also the reason some men develop 'moobs' ('man boobs' or male breasts). So it's good for men to have healthy progesterone levels in order to prevent this conversion of testosterone into dangerous levels of oestradiol.

Progesterone and DHEA, which reduce body fat and keep insulin levels low, can also prevent men from developing a 'middle-aged paunch' (the equivalent of 'middle-aged spread' in women). High insulin levels often lead to an increase in body fat around the tummy.

Too much oestradiol in men is not good but neither is too little. Whereas testosterone builds bone, oestrogen helps to maintain bone. Both hormones are important for male bone health but also for emotional wellbeing. Too much testosterone can cause aggressive and violent behaviour, but these negative traits are generally kept in check by the body's oestrogen levels.

# John's story

## LACK OF STAMINA, EXPANDING WAISTLINE

**The Hormone Doctor:** John was a successful CEO of a small public company. He was 55, in his second marriage and had two young children. I had treated his wife for mild postnatal depression and increasingly severe PMS. John was incredibly smart, and, being muscular and sporty, looked 10 years younger than his age and wanted to stay that way. He had no major complaints except that he'd been feeling more tired than usual and could not play as strenuous a game of tennis as before. He felt that he did not have the stamina and drive he needed for his work, and his vanity had been somewhat injured by the fact that he had started to gain weight around his middle. He came to me because he'd read in a men's magazine that DHEA could help him lose that little bit extra around the waist.

I always carry out blood tests before I treat male patients with either testosterone or DHEA, as I'm acutely aware of the effect these hormones can have on the prostate gland. Before I consider treatment, I always check my patient's PSA (prostate-specific antigen) levels and, if this is elevated, refer him back to his GP to clarify the cause.

In John's case this was not necessary. His constitution was very good, and his blood tests showed that all hormones were in an optimal range – except for DHEA, which was low. I surmised that this could explain John's decreased stamina and expanded waistline, and so prescribed him a daily 50 milligram dose of DHEA. Having already seen a nutritionist, John was taking daily supplements of CoQ10 (important for aerobic cellular respiration and the production of energy in cells) and antioxidants with selenium and zinc, so there was no need to alter his diet.

I saw John every three months for a review of his prescription. His former stamina returned, his tennis game improved and he was even doing his belt up one notch tighter than before he had put on the weight.

Luckily for John, his was a straightforward case. Sadly, for many of my patients the situation is not so clear-cut. As this next case study illustrates, however, complicated medical histories can also have simple solutions. As doctors we need to look at the bigger picture and try to understand what other factors are influencing our patients' health. In treating an illness, we need to know which issues will be easy to solve and which require extensive consideration. This is where patients can become disappointed with their doctors – there are usually no quick fixes. Only in pulling the pieces together – and often this takes a significant amount of time – can doctors form a complete picture of their patient's needs.

## Andrew's story

### ERECTILE DYSFUNCTION, LACK OF STAMINA

**The Hormone Doctor:** Andrew came for his first consultation accompanied by his wife, Jill. Andrew, who was in his early 60s, was tall, strong and well built. He still went surfing every morning and worked as a handyman during the day. He seemed to me to be very masculine but looked a little unhappy when he walked into my clinic.

Men are notorious for avoiding doctors and, in my experience, when they do finally visit a professional they are often reluctant to give details of their ailments. Jill complained that her husband was depressed, did not want to sleep with her any more, and was becoming somewhat of a recluse. He preferred to spend time in his shed listening to music and was only present at mealtimes. He was always up at dawn to go surfing, went to bed early and would usually be fast asleep by the time Jill joined him. Jill was also becoming quite depressed; she felt that their marriage of more than 30 years was coming to an end.

They were both very open about the problems they were having. Andrew told me that it was difficult for him to maintain an erection, and that these days he rarely had morning erections. In fact, he had already been to an impotence clinic and the only solution they offered was Viagra. Although Andrew was fairly healthy, he had developed hypertension a few years earlier and was on medication to control his blood pressure and statins to lower his cholesterol. Viagra was contraindicated with these medications and so wasn't the best choice for his erectile issues. Andrew wanted to understand why he was having these problems for the first time in his life.

Andrew's blood tests confirmed that he had low testosterone and DHEA levels – his testosterone result was in the pre-pubertal range, something no man likes to hear. The blood-pressure medication Andrew was taking is known to cause impotence, which complicated the situation. Low levels of testosterone lead to fewer morning erections; for some men, waking up without their morning glory signals the beginning of the end of their sex life.

I prescribed Andrew a combination of DHEA and testosterone in a lozenge to be taken daily. I also referred him to Vicki, as I felt he needed to take some care with and interest in his nutrition and eating habits.

**The Nutritionist:** I have treated many men like Andrew in my clinic over the years, and it always saddens me to see such seemingly vital men feeling so 'empty' inside. The complication of Andrew's hypertension was the main concern. There are a number of nutritional 'helping hands' for impotence that are contraindicated with hypertension and related medication, so I had to exercise caution.

I recommended that Andrew take Siberian ginseng, a well-known libido enhancer. Ginseng is an adaptogen, which means it can help to stimulate or suppress the function of the adrenal glands, aiding the body's ability to manage stress. Since Andrew's depression was causing him stress, I recommended that he take ginseng daily for three months and proposed to monitor its effects before deciding whether or not he should take it in the long term.

I also suggested that Andrew take ginkgo biloba – a plant extract that helps with blood flow, even on a microcirculation level (to the tiny vessels often at the outer extremities of the body). Ginkgo also benefits the cardiovascular system and brain function. It takes up to two months before the effects of ginkgo are experienced, but Andrew felt that this was a worthwhile investment.

Finally, I prescribed zinc, which has been proven to increase the natural production of testosterone. It's also important for immunity and acts as a natural antidepressant. Andrew was delighted with my suggestion that he eat oysters once a week – their zinc content is unrivalled and their cholesterol levels considerably lower than most other shellfish. I cautioned him, though, about his self-confessed sugar obsession. When it comes to cholesterol, sugar is by far the worst culprit. It is more quickly converted into excess cholesterol than high-cholesterol foods such as shellfish, and sugar has the additional drawback of raising oestrogen levels. Other than this, I couldn't fault Andrew and Jill's diet. Both generally ate in a healthy way, with home-cooked meals made from fresh, often organic food.

Two months later Andrew's mood had improved and his stamina

increased, but he told me that his erectile function still left a lot to be desired.

This is an example of when hormonal supplementation and nutritional advice can't sort it all out. Andrew did feel more comfortable with himself, however, and Jill was pleased that at least he had been willing to acknowledge his problems and attempt to find solutions.

**The Hormone Doctor:** Both Jill and Andrew were pleased with and motivated by Vicki's advice. When Andrew returned to me for a follow-up consultation six weeks later, he confirmed that he was feeling better, his moods were more positive, and that he felt healthier and more energetic.

He said that his libido had increased but admitted he was still having difficulty maintaining an erection for long periods of time. Fortunately, this did not seem to distress him as it had before, and on the whole he was feeling more positive.

I saw Andrew again in another three months and his situation had not changed significantly. His moods were good, his stamina had increased, but his erectile dysfunction had not improved considerably. We discussed this at some length and concluded that his hypertensive medication was contributing to his problems.

In the six months that followed we met regularly so I could monitor Andrew's response to the hormone supplementation and adjust it accordingly. He reported that on some mornings he did wake with an erection, but on the whole his sexual life was not as satisfactory as he and Jill had hoped it might be. Unfortunately, I could only help Andrew partially. Physically and mentally he felt better, but there was no massive improvement in his erectile function. It is often the hope of many men (and women) that testosterone supplementation can solve this problem.

Many factors contribute to erectile dysfunction and there is no quick fix – sometimes there is no fix at all. Every man and couple facing this problem needs to understand this and have realistic expectations of themselves and their partners.

# James's story

## TIRED AND DEPRESSED BUT NO REASONS WHY

**The Hormone Doctor:** When James and his wife Anne arrived in my clinic, the first thing James told me was that he had come only because his wife had made him. She thought he might be depressed and needed a blood test. He thought he was okay.

James, who was in his late 40s, was happy in his job and enjoyed 'switching off' on weekends by playing sport with his cricket-mad son. Anne said James was no longer interested in socialising, that he wanted to spend the weekends at home with his son, and that he watched television endlessly at night and then fell asleep almost immediately without any attempt at intimacy.

Anne missed her husband, the enthusiasm he used to have and the conversations they used to enjoy. James was retreating into his world – work during the week and sports activities on the weekend. Anne said she had started making major decisions about schooling, the house and holidays by herself, as James was not interested in or engaging with her. Anne was becoming a lonely wife and James was withdrawing. He was functioning on a basic level – he was going through the motions – but there seemed to be no sense of vitality or happiness in his life.

James did not want to discuss what was happening. For him it simply was as it was, but Anne insisted on seeking help. James's libido was waning, as were his affection for and interest in his wife.

As James hadn't had a check-up for a long time, I ran some blood tests and checked his general health and hormone profile. James had elevated uric acid levels and had already had one attack of gout in previous years. His cholesterol was mildly elevated, but his blood sugar levels were good, as was his liver function. I checked his thyroid function and that was normal, but his testosterone levels were in the low range of normal and his adrenal-gland hormone DHEA was very low.

Like many men, James resisted the idea of taking pills, but when I explained that 50 milligrams of DHEA daily could help with his energy levels, he was willing to give it a try. I would also have loved to have prescribed him some vitamins but they just weren't his thing.

Taking just a single capsule of DHEA each morning made quite a difference to James's moods and energy. He may have had a sub-clinical depression, but with the DHEA his enthusiasm returned and so did his libido. James had never suffered from erection problems; he simply had lost the desire to have sex.

Anne was thrilled with James's transformation – she felt she had her old husband back. James was more content and became more interested in the world and in people around him.

This is quite a common situation. What is uncommon is that patients do something to get the help they need. Our lives are so much more demanding today, but with supplementation of the hormones that keep us active, we can maintain the lifestyles we want for ourselves.

# resources

**British Association of Nutritional Therapists (BANT)**
www.bant.org.uk

**Complementary Medical Association (CMA)**
www.the-cma.org.uk

**The Doctor's Laboratory (hormone testing blood analysis – doctor's referral only)**
www.tdlpathology.com
020 7307 7383

**British Society for Allergy, Environmental and Nutritional Medicine**
Incorporates the Journal of Nutritional and Environmental Medicine
www.jnem.demon.co.uk

**YorkTest Laboratories (allergy testing)**
www.yorktest.com
0800 074 6185

**Genova Diagnostics Europe Headquarters (digestive and toxic testing)**
www.gdx.uk.net
020 8336 7751


## NUTRIENT SUPPLIERS
**The Nutri Centre (supplies most brands manufactured in the USA and UK, as well as herbal remedies and superfood powders)**
www.nutricentre.com
020 7637 8436 – mail order

**Nutri-Link (supplies nutritional supplements, blood type testing kits, seminars and workshops)**
www.nutri-linkltd.co.uk
0874 054 002

**Biocare (British manufacturers of superior nutritional supplements, training seminars)**
www.biocare.co.uk
0121 433 3727

**Oxford Medical Supplies (China Med range of high quality Chinese herbs)**
www.oxfordmedical.co.uk
0800 975 8000

## ORGANIC FOOD AGENCIES
**The Soil Association (advising on all criteria relating to organic produce)**
www.soilassociation.org

**Organic Food Directory (lists all suppliers throughout Britain, Wales, Scotland and Ireland)**
www.organicfood.co.uk

**The Food Standards Agency (Government regulatory body for Food Health and Safety)**
www.food.gov.uk

## ORGANIC FOOD BOX DELIVERIES
**Abel and Cole (countrywide – UK)**
www.abelandcole.co.uk

**Riverford Organics (countrywide – UK)**
www.riverfordorganicveg.co.uk

**Wholefoods Organic Food Emporium (world's largest retailer of organic produce and products for the home – London and North America)**
www.wholefoodsmarket.com

**Borough Market (London's oldest organic open-air market selling produce from all over Britain)**
www.boroughmarket.org.uk

## COMPOUNDING PHARMACIES
### The Specialist Pharmacy
42 Windmill Street
London W1T 2JX
+44 (0) 207 637 1055
www.specialist-pharmacy.com

A bespoke independent pharmacy specialising in individually prescribed
hormone prescriptions and vitamin supplements for health and beauty.


## ADDITIONAL READING
Glenville, Marilyn, *New Natural Alternatives to HRT*, Kyle Cathie, London, 2003.
——, *Eat Your Way through the Menopause*, Kyle Cathie, London, 2002.
Kearns, Linda, *Eat to Beat the Menopause*, Thorsons, 2002.
Love, Susan, and Lindsey, Karen, *Dr. Susan Love's Hormone Book,* Random
    House, USA, 1997.
——, *Dr. Susan Love's Breast Book,* Perseus, 2004.
Northrup, Christiane, *The Wisdom of Menopause: Creating Physical and
    Emotional Health and Healing During the Change*, Bantam Books, New York,
    2006.
——, *Women's Bodies, Women's Wisdom: Creating Physical and Emotional Health
    and Healing*, Bantam Books, New York, 2006.
Smith, Pamela Wartian, *HRT: The Answers*, Healthy Living Books, Traverse City,
    2003.
Reiss, Uzzi, *Natural Hormone Balance for Women: Look Younger, Feel Stronger,
    and Live Life with Exuberance*, Pocket Books, New York, 2001.
Tan, Robert S., *The Andropause Mystery: Unraveling Truths about the Male
    Menopause*, AMRED Publishing, Houston, 2001.
Teaff, Nancy Lee, *Perimenopause: Preparing for the Change*, Prima Publishing,
    US, 2003.


## SCIENTIFIC PAPERS TO SHOW YOUR DOCTOR
### HRT and oral contraceptive pill cancer risk
Anon. (2006), 'Saving the innocents: a journey to the source to say "neigh" to
    Premarin', *Townsend Letter: The Examiner of Alternative Medicine*, November
    issue.
Beral, V. & Million Women Study Collaborators (2003), 'Breast cancer and
    hormone-replacement therapy in the Million Women Study', *Lancet*
    362(9382), pp. 419–27.
Campagnoli, C., Clavel-Chapelon, F., Kaaks, R. *et al.* (2005), 'Progestins and

progesterone in hormone replacement therapy and the risk of breast cancer', *Journal of Steroid Biochemistry and Molecular Biology* 96(2), pp. 95–108.

Canfell, K., Banks E., Moa, A.M. & Beral, V. (2008), 'Decrease in breast cancer incidence following a rapid fall in use of hormone replacement therapy in Australia', *Medical Journal of Australia* 188(11), pp. 641–44.

Chlebowski, R.T., Kuller, L.H., Prentice, R.L. *et al.* (2009), 'Breast cancer after use of estrogen plus progestin in postmenopausal women', *New England Journal of Medicine* 360(6), pp. 573–87.

Goodwin, P.J., Ennis, M., Pritchard, K.I. *et al.* (2009) 'Prognostic effects of 25-hydroxyvitamin D levels in early breast cancer', *Journal of Clinical Oncology* 27(23), pp. 3757–63.

Kumle, M., Weiderpass, E., Braaten, T. *et al.* (2002), 'Use of oral contraceptives and breast cancer risk: The Norwegian–Swedish Women's Lifestyle and Health cohort study', *Cancer Epidemiology, Biomarkers & Prevention* 11(11), pp. 1375–81.

Lund, E., Bakken, K., Dumeaux, V. *et al.* (2007), 'Hormone replacement therapy and breast cancer in former users of oral contraceptives – The Norwegian Women and Cancer study', *International Journal of Cancer* 121(3), pp. 645–48.

## Mammogram risk

Gøtzsche, P.C. & Olsen, O. (2000), 'Is screening for breast cancer with mammography justifiable?', *Lancet* 355(9198), pp. 129–34.

## Oestrogen metabolism

Bradlow, H.L., Telang, N.T., Sepkovic, D.W. & Osborne, M.P. (1996), '2-hydroxyestrone: the "good" estrogen', *Journal of Endocrinology* 150, pp. S259–65.

Head, K. (1998), 'Estriol: safety and efficacy', *Alternative Medicine Review* 3(2), pp. 101–13.

Miller, K. (2003), 'Estrogen and DNA damage: the silent source of breast cancer?' *Journal of the National Cancer Institute* 95(2), pp. 100–102.

Muti, P., Westerlind, K., Wu, T. *et al.* (2002), 'Urinary estrogen metabolites and prostate cancer: a case–control study in the United States', *Cancer Causes Control* 13(10), pp. 947–55.

Risbridger, G.P., Ellem, S.J. & McPherson, S.J. (2007), 'Estrogen action on the prostate gland: a critical mix of endocrine and paracrine signaling', *Journal of Molecular Endocrinology* 39(3), pp. 183–88.

Rogan, E.G., Badawi, A.F., Devanesan, P.D. *et al.* (2003), 'Relative imbalances in estrogen metabolism and conjugation in breast tissue of women with carcinoma: potential biomarkers of susceptibility to cancer', *Carcinogenesis* 24(4), pp. 697–702.

Sarkar, F.H. & Li, Y. (2009), 'Harnessing the fruits of nature for the development of multi-targeted cancer therapeutics', *Cancer Treatment Reviews* 35(7), pp. 597–607.

Zeligs, M.A. (2008) 'Prostate health promotion with diindolylmethane (DIM)', The Doctor's Research Update: Natural Medicine for Men's Health, dimfaq. com/index.htm, accessed 1 May 2008.

Zeligs, M.A. (1999), 'Safer estrogen with phytonutrition', *Townsend Letter for Doctors and Patients* 189(April), pp. 83–88.

## Nutrition and oestrogen clearance

Goldin, B.R., Adlercreutz, H., Dwyer, J.T. *et al.* (1981), 'Effect of diet on excretion of estrogens in pre- and postmenopausal women', *Cancer Research* 41(9 Part 2), pp. 3771–73.

Lord, R.S., Bongiovanni, B., & Bralley, J.A. (2002), 'Estrogen metabolism and the diet–cancer connection: rationale for assessing the ratio of urinary hydroxylated estrogen metabolites', *Alternative Medicine Review* 7(2), pp. 112–29.

## Bioavailable diindolylmethane (DIM)

Dalessandri, K.M., Firestone, K.M., Firestone, G.L., Fitch, M.D. *et al.* (2004), 'Pilot study: effect of 3,3'-diindolylmethane supplements on urinary hormone metabolites in postmenopausal women with a history of early-stage breast cancer', *Nutrition and Cancer* 50(2), pp. 161–67.

Sarkar, F.H. & Li, Y. (2009), 'Harnessing the fruits of nature for the development of multi-targeted cancer therapeutics', *Cancer Treatment Reviews* 35(7), pp. 597–607.

Zeligs, M.A., Sepkovic, D.W., Manrique, C. *et al.* (2002), 'Absorption-enhanced 3,3'-diindolylmethane: human use in HPV-related, benign and pre-cancerous conditions', *Proceedings of the American Association for Cancer Research* 43, p. 3198.

## Indole-3-carbinol

Bradlow, H.L. (2008), 'Indole-3-carbinol as a chemoprotective agent in breast and prostate cancer', *In Vivo* 22, pp. 441–46.

Zeligs, M.A. (2001), 'The cruciferous choice: diindolylmethane or I3C?: Phytonutrient supplements for cancer prevention and health promotion', *Townsend Letter for Doctors and Patients* 217(August), pp. 47–53.

## Xenoestrogens and health risks

Brody, J.G. & Rudel, R.A. (2008), 'Environmental pollutants and breast cancer: the evidence from animal and human studies', *Breast Diseases: A Year Book Quarterly*, 19(1), pp. 17–19.

Charlier, C. & Dejardine, M.-T.C. (2007) 'Increased risk of relapse after breast cancer with exposure to organochlorine pollutants', *Bulletin of Environmental Contamination and Toxicology* 78(1), pp. 1–4.

Charlier, C., Albert, A., Herman, P. *et al.* (2003), 'Breast cancer and serum organochlorine residues', *Occupational and Environmental Medicine* 60(5), pp. 348–51.

Cohn, B.A., Wolff, M.S., Cirillo, P.M. *et al.* (2007), 'DDT and breast cancer in young women: new data on the significance of age at exposure', *Environmental Health Perspectives* 115(10), pp. 1406–14.

Crisp, T.M., Clegg, E.D., Cooper, R.L. *et al.* (1998), 'Environmental endocrine disruption: an effects assessment and analysis', *Environmental Health Perspectives* 106(S1), pp. 11–56.

Diamanti-Kandarakis, E., Bourguignon, J.P., Giudice, L.C. *et al.* (2009), 'Endocrine-disrupting chemicals: an Endocrine Society scientific statement', *Endocrine Reviews* 30(4), pp. 293–342.

Gray, J., Evans, N., Taylor, B. *et al.* (2009), 'State of the evidence: the connection between breast cancer and the environment', *International Journal of Occupational and Environmental Health*, 15(1), pp. 43–78.

Kortenkamp, A. (2008), 'Breast cancer and exposure to hormonally active chemicals: an appraisal of the scientific evidence', Centre for Toxicology, School of Pharmacy, University of London, UK, chemicalshealthmonitor.org/spip.php?rubrique100, accessed 1 May 2008.

McElroy, J.A., Egan, K.M., Titus-Ernstoff, L. *et al.* (2007) 'Occupational exposure to electromagnetic field and breast cancer risk in a large, population-based, case-control study in the United States', *Journal of Occupational and Environmental Medicine* 49(3), pp. 266–74.

Michnovicz, J.J. & Galbraith, R.A. (1991), 'Cimetidine inhibits catechol estrogen metabolism in women', *Metabolism* 40(2), pp. 170–74.

Prins, G.S. (2008), 'Endocrine disruptors and prostate cancer risk', *Endocrine-Related Cancer* 15(3), pp. 649–56.

Safe, S.H. (1995), 'Environmental and dietary estrogens and human health: is there a problem?', *Environmental Health Perspectives* 103(4), pp. 346–51.

Sasco, A.J. (2001), 'Epidemiology of breast cancer: an environmental disease?', *APMIS: Acta Pathologica, Microbiologica et Immunologica Scandinavica* 109(5), pp. 321–32.

Sultan, C., Balaguer, P. & Terouanne, B. (2001), 'Environmental xenoestrogens, antiandrogens and disorders of male sexual differentiation', *Molecular and Cell Endocrinology* 178(1–2), pp. 99–105.

## Diethylstilbestrol (DES): synthetic oestrogen exposure

Palmer, J.R., Wise, L.A., Hatch, E.E. *et al.* (2006), 'Prenatal diethylstilbestrol exposure and risk of breast cancer', *Cancer Epidemiology, Biomarkers & Prevention* 15(8), pp. 1509–14.

Park, S.K., Kang, D., McGlynn, K.A. *et al.* (2008), 'Intrauterine environments and breast cancer risk: meta-analysis and systematic review', *Breast Cancer Research* 10(1), pp. R8.

## Obesity and hormone balance

Abate, N., Haffner, S.M., Garg, A. *et al.* (2002), 'Sex steroid hormones, upper body obesity, and insulin resistance', *Journal of Clinical Endocrinology & Metabolism* 87(10), pp. 4522–27.

Barnard, R.J. (2007), 'Prostate cancer prevention by nutritional means to alleviate metabolic syndrome', *American Journal of Clinical Nutrition* 86(3), pp. 889S–93S.

Cooke, P.S. & Naaz, A. (2004), 'Role of estrogens in adipocyte development and function', Minireview. *Experimental Biology and Medicine* 229, pp. 1127–35.

Harvie, M., Hooper, L. & Howell, A.H. (2003), 'Central obesity and breast cancer risk: a systematic review', *Obesity Research* 4(3), pp. 157–73.

Hershcopf, R.J. & Bradlow, H.L. (1987) 'Obesity, diet, endogenous estrogens, and the risk of hormone-sensitive cancer', *American Journal of Clinical Nutrition* 45(1), pp. 283–89.

McTiernan, A. (2003), 'Behavioral risk factors in breast cancer: can risk be modified?' *The Oncologist* 8(4), pp. 326–34.

Schneider, J. (1983), 'Effects of obesity on estradiol metabolism: decreased formation of nonuterotropic metabolites', *Journal of Clinical Endocrinology & Metabolism* 56(5), pp. 973–78.

# WEB RESOURCES

## Useful sites

Breast Cancer Action: bcaction.org
Contaminated Without Consent: ej4all.org/contaminatedwithoutconsent
Dr Michael Murray: doctormurray.com
Life Extension Foundation: lef.org
Natural News: naturalnews.com
Our Stolen Future: ourstolenfuture.org/index.htm
Science and Environmental Health Network: sehn.org
Silent Spring Institute: silentspring.org
Skin Deep: Cosmetic Safety Database: cosmeticsdatabase.com
Vitamin D Council: vitamindcouncil.org
The Women's Health Initiative (WHI) Study: whi.org

# index